Near Misses in Pulmonary and Cardiothoracic Critical Care

Near Misses in Pulmonary and Cardiothoracic Critical Care

Joseph Varon, M.D., F.A.C.P., F.C.C.P., F.C.C.M.

Assistant Professor of Medicine, Pulmonary and Critical Care Section, Baylor College of Medicine, Houston; Research Director, Department of Emergency Medicine, The Methodist Hospital, Houston

Garrett L. Walsh, M.D., M.Sc., F.R.C.S.C., F.A.C.S., F.C.C.M.

Associate Professor of Surgery, Department of Thoracic and Cardiovascular Surgery, and Associate Professor of Critical Care, The University of Texas, M. D. Anderson Cancer Center, Houston

Robert E. Fromm, Jr., M.D., M.P.H., F.A.C.P., F.C.C.P., F.C.C.M.

Associate Professor of Medicine, Sections of Cardiology and Pulmonary and Critical Care, Baylor College of Medicine, Houston; Director, Emergency Services, The Methodist Hospital, Houston

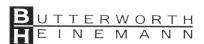

Boston   Oxford   Auckland   Johannesburg   Melbourne   New Delhi

Library of Congress Cataloging-in-Publication Data

Near misses in pulmonary and cardiothoracic critical care / edited by
    Joseph Varon, Garrett L. Walsh, Robert E. Fromm, Jr.
        p. cm.
    Includes bibliographical references and index.
    ISBN 0-7506-7117-3
    1. Cardiac intensive care--Case studies. 2. Respiratory intensive
care--Case studies. I. Varon, Joseph. II. Walsh, Garrett L.
III. Fromm, Robert E.
    [DNLM: 1. Lung Diseases case studies. 2. Heart Diseases case
studies. 3. Critical Care. 4. Medical Errors.   WF 600 N354 1999]
RC684.C36N43   1999
616.1'2028--dc21
DNLM/DLC
for Library of Congress   98-54232
                                                            CIP

British Library Cataloguing-in-Publication Data
A catalogue record for this book is available from the British Library.

The publisher offers special discounts on bulk orders of this book.
For information, please contact:

Manager of Special Sales
Butterworth–Heinemann
225 Wildwood Avenue
Woburn, MA 01801-2041
Tel: 781-904-2500
Fax: 781-904-2620

For information on all Butterworth–Heinemann publications available,
contact our World Wide Web home page at: http://www.bh.com

10 9 8 7 6 5 4 3 2 1

Printed in the United States of America

To the residents and fellows who have inspired us to write this book

Contents

Preface

To many, the definition of critical care is, in fact, a near-disaster or near-catastrophe. However, in this book we illustrate clinical critical care conditions and situations in which errors in *diagnosis or treatment* or *unusual presentations* led to potentially serious consequences. Although some of the situations surrounding these cases may be amusing, our intent in presenting them is entirely serious. The small details in the patient's history and in the technical procedures often can make the difference between life and serious morbidity or death.

This book was written for everyone engaged in critical care medicine, pulmonary medicine, cardiology, and cardiothoracic surgery. We have presented both basic and generally accepted standards of clinical practices, as well as our own opinions, in each of the cases. The cases are presented in no particular order. The case titles hint at the content of the cases without revealing the diagnosis. The references included were intentionally limited, but they provide a reasonable starting point for those interested in more detailed discussion of the issues raised in each case.

Medicine is not a static field; it changes every day. This book is not meant to define the standard of care; instead, it offers general guidelines to current diagnosis and therapy. We hope readers will benefit from our experiences and avert their own near-disasters and near-catastrophes in critical care.

Joseph Varon
Garrett L. Walsh
Robert E. Fromm, Jr.

Near Misses in Pulmonary and Cardiothoracic Critical Care

1

The Bank Robber with a Short Sprint but a Long Lace

Sam is a career criminal with several arrests over the past decade for breaking and entering. He has been out on parole for more than 6 months but, unfortunately, has decided to return to the world of crime. Sam has been staking out a small bank for more than 2 weeks, planning in great detail all of the maneuvers that he must execute in the heist.

On the morning of the robbery, he steals a car with handicapped license plates, drives to the bank, and parks the car in a designated handicapped spot less than 50 feet from the entrance. The car is left idling, with the driver's door unlocked. He feigns a limp and slowly but calmly joins the line of bank patrons waiting to deposit their checks. He pretends to fill out a deposit slip. When his turn comes, he quietly passes the teller the deposit slip, on which the words "Give me all the money. I have a gun" are written in block letters. The teller is caught by surprise but composes herself and quickly loads the duffle bag that he has passed to her with money. While packing the bag, and without Sam's noticing, she activates a silent bank alarm with her left foot. A police cruiser one block away receives the radio dispatch and accelerates toward the bank. Once the duffel bag has been filled, Sam rushes for the front entrance.

Just as Sam exits the building, a police car comes around the corner. Sam draws his revolver and bolts for his idling getaway car, but in his haste he trips on a shoelace and falls to the pavement. He gets up again. The police, now in range, order him to stop. Sam points his revolver and at once is shot in the left chest in the anterior axillary line at the level of the fifth intercostal space. He falls to the pavement. The police disarm him, and an ambulance is called to transport him to the level I trauma center.

On his arrival at the hospital, Sam is conscious but tachycardic; his pulse is 130 bpm and systolic blood pressure is 70 mm Hg. He has a solitary entrance wound without an exit wound. He has diminished breath sounds on the left with a normal right chest examination, a normal cardiac examination, and no elevation of his jugular venous pressure. An abdominal examination is normal. He has full range of motion in all four limbs and denies any neurologic symptoms.

Large-bore intravenous (IV) lines are started, and a left chest tube is placed. More than 2 liters of blood is evacuated, and he continues to have ongoing bleeding. He is rapidly transfused with O– blood and transported immediately to the surgical suites for an emergency left thoracotomy.

Sam is stable on induction and rapidly placed in a right lateral decubitus position. His chest is opened through a standard posterolateral thoracotomy through the fifth intercostal space. On opening the chest, a large hemothorax is evacuated. Significant bleeding is noted from an intercostal artery and a damaged portion of the superior segment of the left lower lobe. The artery is suture-ligated, and a gastrointestinal anastomosis stapler is used to remove the destroyed portion of the left lower lobe. Once the bleeding is controlled, a concerted effort is made to locate the bullet. The bullet can be tracked posteriorly where it missed the aorta and esophagus, but it appears to have come to rest in the paravertebral soft tissues, and the portable chest radiograph seems to suggest a midline position. The bullet cannot be located but is presumed to be in the paravertebral musculature (Figure 1-1). When the bleeding is under control, the chest is closed.

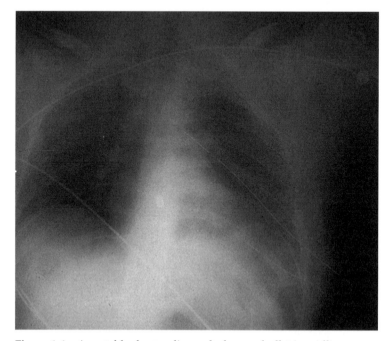

Figure 1-1 A portable chest radiograph shows a bullet in midline.

While in the intensive care unit (ICU), Sam recovers and improves quickly. Forty-eight hours later, he is ready to be transferred to the floor, but requires constant police supervision. He complains of some leg numbness while walking through the wards. A computed tomographic (CT) scan is performed to accurately evaluate the position of the bullet and see whether it is contributing to this new neurologic symptom. The CT scan (Figure 1-2) reveals the incredible position of the bullet: in the spinal canal, parallel to the spinal cord. A posterior laminectomy is performed to remove the bullet. His neurologic symptoms normalize after the procedure.

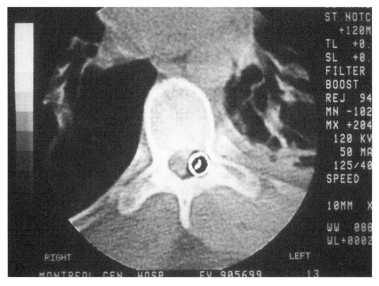

Figure 1-2 Computed tomography shows a bullet in the spinal canal, lying next to the spinal cord.

DISCUSSION

Management of gunshot wounds is complex and varies depending on the trajectory and course of the bullet and the caliber of the weapon. Although entrance and exit wounds may exist, they do not necessarily predict a straight-line passage of the bullet, which can ricochet and cause significant damage.

In this case, advanced trauma life support was appropriately employed. A drainage of more than 1,000 ml on initial placement of the chest tube was, in this as in every case, grounds for immediate thoracotomy. The choice between standard thoracotomy or sternotomy using a clamshell incision depends on which procedure permits best access to the organs of the chest. Injuries to the lung can often be managed with pulmonary resection using stapling devices. A host of serious injuries can occur, including injury to the heart and great vessels that occasionally presents with exsanguinating hemorrhage (although hemorrhage may also be delayed). Other structures at risk include the esophagus, the diaphragm, and even the spinal cord. Isolated injuries to the thoracic duct have been described; unless bleeding is initially high or persistent, a chest tube is often all that is required for the management of such patients. Prolonged air leaks and empyema can complicate these injuries. This case is remarkable because the patient presented with no neurologic symptoms but worsened over a 48- to 72-hour period.

CLINICAL POINTS TO REMEMBER

1. The management of gunshot wounds is complex and varies depending on the trajectory and course of the bullet and the caliber of the weapon.
2. In gunshot injuries to the chest, a drainage of more than 1,000 ml on initial placement of the chest tube is grounds for immediate thoracotomy.
3. Prolonged air leaks and empyema can complicate these injuries.

SELECTED READINGS

Bilsker MS, Bauerlein EJ, Kamerman ML. Bullet embolus from the heart to the right subclavian artery after gunshot wound to the right chest. Am Heart J 1996;132:1093–1094.

Inci I, Ozcelik C, Nizam O, et al. Penetrating chest injuries in children: a review of 94 cases. J Ped Surg 1996;31:673–676.

Kennedy FR, Cornwell EE, Camel J, et al. Aorto-esophageal fistulae due to gunshot wounds: report of two cases with one survivor. J Trauma 1995;38:971–974.

Petricevic A, Ilic N, Bacic A, et al. War injuries of the lungs. Eur J Cardiothorac Surg 1997;11:843–847.

Worthington MG, de Groot M, Gunning AJ, von Oppell UO. Isolated thoracic duct injury after penetrating chest trauma. Ann Thorac Surg 1995;60:272–274.

2

The Wealthy Man with a Bloody Cough

Bill is a 43-year-old businessman who has been traveling across the world promoting one of his new products. Late one Saturday evening, Bill returns from the Fiji Islands and begins to have nonproductive coughing. While driving his new Ferrari, he has a coughing spell that prevents him from driving. This time the cough produces white sputum with a little blood. He calls his high-profile physician, Dr. Jones, who instructs him to come to the office on Monday for a tuberculosis test because Bill has been flying through many Third World countries. Bill goes to a local pharmacy to buy a cough suppressant; he feels better after taking the syrup and, believing that his chances of having tuberculosis are minimal, does not see his physician that week. Bill's symptoms improve, and he continues to work in his usual fashion.

Two weeks later, after clearing customs from an overseas flight, Bill is seen in an emergency department (ED) with chest pain and massive hemoptysis. Bill tells the local physicians that he has had occasional expectoration of minimal amounts of blood for 2 weeks. On the day of admission, he has pleuritic chest pain and coughs up more than 500 ml of bright red blood. Bill's medical, surgical, and family histories are not significant for tuberculosis, tobacco use, cardiovascular or pulmonary diseases, or previous operations.

A chest radiograph obtained on arrival at the ED demonstrates a possible infiltrate in the right upper lobe (Figure 2-1). Bill is admitted to the hospital for further diagnostic workup and observation, where a chest CT study (Figure 2-2) reveals a mass in the anterior mediastinum and an irregular infiltrate in the anterior segment of the right upper lobe. A CT-guided fine-needle aspiration of the mass reveals only epithelial cells. Fiberoptic bronchoscopy fails to demonstrate any endobronchial pathology or active sites of bleeding. Because the patient remains hemodynamically stable during hospitalization and has no further episodes of hemoptysis, he is discharged and instructed to follow up with his personal physician.

Bill returns to his home and immediately calls Dr. Jones, who asks him to come to the office as soon as possible. Bill has an important meeting that day, as always, and cannot go to Dr.

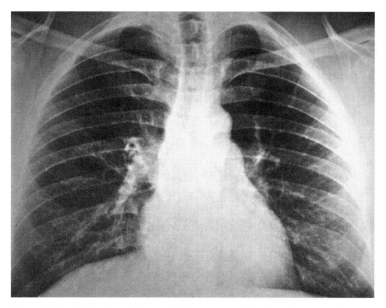

Figure 2-1   A chest radiograph taken on admission shows a discrete infiltrate in the right upper lobe.

Jones' office. That evening, in the middle of his business meeting, Bill has another episode of hemoptysis and is rushed to the hospital. On arriving at the ED, he indicates that he had recurrent hemoptysis of approximately 700 ml of blood during the meeting and another 400 ml in the ambulance and on presentation to the ED. Vital signs on arrival at the ED include blood pressure of 120/90 mm Hg, heart rate of 112 bpm, and respiratory rate of 30 breaths per minute. He is able to maintain his airway by coughing.

Bill is taken directly to the operating room, where bronchoscopy reveals active bleeding from the right upper lobe. An 8-Fr Fogarty catheter is inserted to block the right upper lobe bronchus and protect the remaining tracheobronchial tree. A median sternotomy is performed. A bilobulate mass in the anterior mediastinum, involving the right upper lobe, is identified. An en bloc resection of the mass with thymic tissue, pericardium, and a nonanatomic wedge of the right upper lobe is performed using a stapling device. The mass had directly invaded the right upper lobe and the right internal mammary artery, which required ligation. The invasion of this large systemic artery likely accounts for the massive bright red bleeding. Final pathology shows a mature mediastinal teratoma, probably arising in the thymus, with old hemorrhage and surround-

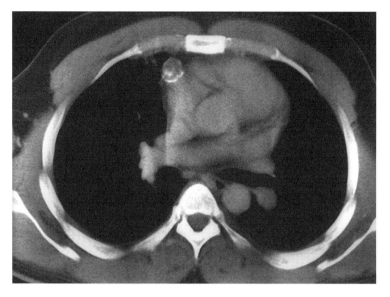

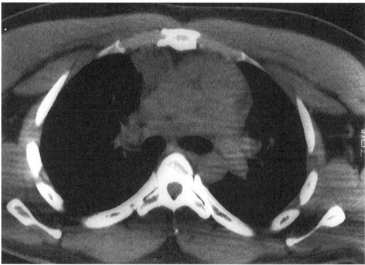

Figure 2-2 Computed tomography of the chest reveals a mass lesion on the right side in the anterior mediastinum. The lesion shows areas of calcification and is adjacent to the right upper lobe of the lung.

ing fibrosis and calcifications. No evidence of immature elements or other germ cell components is found. Bill is discharged 1 week later. On a follow-up visit, he is improving rapidly and approaching his baseline functional status, with no further recurrence of hemoptysis. From now on, he will be compliant with his appointments.

DISCUSSION

Massive hemoptysis is commonly defined as expectoration of more than 600 ml of blood per 24 hours in an adult. Hemoptysis has been described in more than 100 different disease processes; the most common are listed in Table 2-1. It is rare, however, that a benign mediastinal teratoma presents with massive hemoptysis.

There are few reports in the literature of patients with teratoma whose initial presentation is hemoptysis. Hayden et al. describe a patient with hemoptysis due to a benign intrathoracic teratoma that caused systemic-pulmonary artery shunting. They report that bleeding was caused at least in part by extensive pleural adhesions. Kakkar et al. describe a patient with a primary pulmonary malignant teratoma with yolk sac elements that was associated with myelofibrosis and presented with hemoptysis. Steier reports a patient with recurrent hemoptysis who was found at thoracotomy to have a benign intrapulmonary cystic teratoma. Morgan published a case report and review of the literature about intrapulmonary teratomas; although all of the patients with benign and malignant teratomas had hemoptysis on presentation, none of them had massive hemoptysis as in Bill's case.

Primary germ cell tumors account for 10% of mediastinal tumors in adults. Only 1% of germ cell tumors are found in the mediastinum; the vast majority originate in the gonads or the retroperitoneum. Mediastinal teratomas are nonseminomatous primary germ cell tumors. Benign mediastinal teratomas (dermoid cysts) are seen with equal frequency in women and men, unlike malignant teratomas, which are much more common in men. The histology shows tissue such as skin, hair follicles, cartilage, smooth muscle, and other well-represented organs originating from the endoderm, the ectoderm, and the mesoderm.

In patients presenting with hemoptysis, maintenance of a patent airway is paramount. The patient's oxygenation should be followed and supplemental oxygen provided as indicated. If the bleeding side is known, the patient should be positioned with that side down to prevent spillover to the nonbleeding side. Ideally, if the patient is able to maintain the airway by coughing, intubation should be delayed until the patient has been transported to the operating room, where rigid and flexible bronchoscopy can be performed under optimal conditions.

In cases of impending asphyxiation, the airway should be protected by endotracheal intubation. Viable options are the use of a double-lumen tube to separate the left and the right lung and the use of a Uni-vent tube or endobronchial blocker to prevent spillover. With a double-lumen endobronchial tube, both lungs can be separately ventilated, but insertion and positioning may be very difficult and time-consuming. If it is impossible to place an endobronchial tube, a regular single-lumen endotracheal tube (internal diameter 8.5–9.5 mm) can be advanced for bronchial ventilation to separate the lungs and prevent spillover (assuming the pathologic process is limited to one side). These patients require adequate large-bore peripheral or central IV access, and volume resuscitation should be performed as indicated by the clinical picture and laboratory studies.

An immediate thoracic surgical consultation is required, because most cases need operative intervention for definitive treatment. Expectant medical management of surgical causes of hemoptysis results in significant mortality. Every effort should be made to determine the cause of the hemoptysis. Unfortunately, some underlying diseases that cause hemoptysis are not amenable to surgical resection. These include disseminated

Table 2-1   Diseases most commonly associated with massive hemoptysis

Aspergillomas
Bronchial adenomas
Bronchiectasis
Bronchogenic carcinoma or metastatic cancer
Broncholithiasis
Cystic fibrosis
Immune complex–mediated vasculitis (i.e., Goodpasture's syndrome)
Lung abscess
Pulmonary embolism
Trauma
Tuberculosis

carcinomatosis, advanced extensive bilateral pulmonary disease, and diffuse vasculitis producing hemoptysis (i.e., Goodpasture's syndrome). Operative intervention is also not indicated if the source of bleeding cannot be established or pulmonary function is severely impaired.

In selected patients, embolization of the bleeding vessel with Gelfoam after pulmonary or bronchial angiography may be a treatment option. Because recurrence is quite common, this procedure is used either as a temporizing measure to stabilize patients before an operation or as palliation in patients who are not candidates for surgical intervention.

CLINICAL POINTS TO REMEMBER

1. In patients presenting with hemoptysis, maintenance of a patent airway is paramount.
2. In cases of impending asphyxiation, the airway should be protected by endotracheal intubation.
3. An immediate thoracic surgical consultation is required as most cases require operative intervention for definitive treatment.
4. Mediastinal teratomas are rare tumors that can present with hemoptysis.

SELECTED READINGS

Conlan AA, Hurwitz SS, Krige L, et al. Massive hemoptysis: review of 123 cases. J Thorac Cardiovasc Surg 1983;85:120–124.

Garzon AA, Cerruti MM, Golding ME. Exsanguinating hemoptysis. J Thorac Cardiovasc Surg 1982;84:829–833.

Hayden CK Jr, Swischuk LE, Schwartz MZ, Davis M. Systemic-pulmonary shunting and hemoptysis in a benign intrathoracic teratoma. Pediatr Radiol 1984;14:52–54.

Kakkar N, Vasishta RK, Banerjee AK, et al. Primary pulmonary malignant teratoma with yolk sac element associated with hematologic neoplasia. Respiration 1996;63:52–54.

McCollum WB, Mattox KL, Guinn GA, et al. Immediate operative treatment for massive hemoptysis. Chest 1975;67:152–155.

Morgan DE, Sanders C, McElvein RB, et al. Intrapulmonary teratoma: a case report and review of the literature. J Thorac Imaging 1992;7:70–77.

Robertson JM, Fee HJ, Mulder DG. Mediastinal teratoma causing life-threatening hemoptysis. Its occurrence in an infant. Am J Dis Child 1981;135:148–150.

Steier KJ. Benign cystic teratoma of the lung. Postgrad Med 1988;83:85–86.

Sternbach G, Varon J. Initial evaluation and management of massive hemoptysis. Hosp Physician 1995;31:10–14.

Winter SM, Ingbar DH. Massive hemoptysis: pathogenesis and management. J Intensive Care Med 1988;3:171–188.

3

Chest Pain in a College Party Animal

Jim is a bright, energetic, and athletic undergraduate biology student who has just completed a grueling 2 weeks of final examinations. He has been studying night and day in an attempt to obtain good marks because he plans to apply for medical school next year during his final year of college. After the final papers have been turned in, Jim and his premed buddies decide to celebrate before returning home to start their respective summer jobs. They head straight for the university pub; several pitchers of beers are ordered, and a chug-a-lug contest begins.

After several hours of drinking, they decide to go out and get something to eat and walk down the street to a popular pizzeria. Jim has a large pizza almost entirely to himself. Then they happily stagger down the street, singing the school song, into a local pub, where another round of drinks is ordered. Shortly thereafter Jim starts to feel nauseated and works his way to the rest room, where he has uncontrollable retching and vomits violently several times. During the fourth emetic episode, he develops severe epigastric and left-sided chest pain and loses consciousness transiently. When he comes to, he has a sharp pain in his left chest and shoulder tip that has a pleuritic component to it. At this time a buddy appears at the bathroom door and immediately recognizes that Jim appears cyanotic and acutely ill. Emergency medical services are called.

On arriving at the ED, Jim is tachypneic to 35 bpm and tachycardic to 140 bpm, and his temperature has spiked to 39.6°C. He has developed crepitus in the tissues of his neck. A chest radiograph is performed and reveals a large left-sided pleural effusion. Immediately, a chest tube is placed and several pieces of what appears to be semidigested pieces of pepperoni are drained. A Gastrografin swallow is performed to identify the extent of the injury to the esophagus (Figure 3-1). An emergency thoracic surgical consult is obtained, and surgery is performed after fluid resuscitation and antibiotic administration have been done.

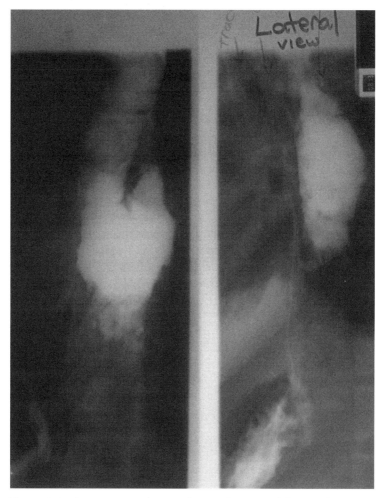

Figure 3-1 A contrast study reveals a perforation of the esophagus.

DISCUSSION

Postemetic rupture of the esophagus was first described in 1724 by Dr. Boerhaave, who recognized it as the cause of death in the Baron van Wassenaer, Grand Admiral of the Fleet of Holland, who would voluntarily induce vomiting after a large meal to purge his stomach to permit further binge eating.

Vomiting is a complicated physiologic mechanism, controlled through the vomiting center in the brain in the floor of the fourth ventricle and the sensory nucleus of the vagus nerve. It requires coordination between voluntary abdominal and chest muscles and the involuntary smooth muscles of the stomach and esophagus. Forceful vomiting against a closed cricopharyngeus muscle can acutely increase the pressure in the esophagus, which can then develop a longitudinal tear in the weakest part of the lower third of its length, with rupture into the left hemithorax almost 80% of the time. This is similar to the rupture of a balloon that is tied at one end while significant pressure is applied to the other end.

The clinical presentation described above is classic for a ruptured esophagus with shoulder tip pain referred from diaphragmatic irritation and subcutaneous emphysema from swallowed air tracking along the mediastinal tissue planes into the neck. Other conditions, including pancreatitis, cholecystitis, peptic ulcer, a vascular event such as aortic dissection, and mesenteric thrombosis may be included in the differential diagnosis.

Boerhaave's syndrome represents a thoracic surgical emergency. Patients in whom the diagnosis is correctly made and the esophagus repaired within 24 hours have a mortality rate of 12%. Mortality is tripled if the diagnosis is unrecognized and surgical repair is delayed 24 hours or longer. Surgery requires identification of the tear or tears and primary repair in two layers. The left chest is the usual approach for lower-third esophageal tears; a right thoracotomy is performed for the occasional tear in the midesophagus. Autologous tissues including thickened parietal pleura, intercostal muscle or diaphragm muscle pedicle flaps, stomach, and pericardium are usually interposed over the repair to aid in healing—esophageal tissues become extremely friable because of the secondary mediastinitis that rapidly develops after repair. The entered mediastinum and chest cavity must be thoroughly lavaged and drained to minimize the chances of the development of postperforation empyema.

When the diagnosis is delayed for 24 hours or more, primary repair of the esophagus may not be possible. Empyema drainage and proximal exclusion techniques that divert the esophageal flow with a cervical esophagostomy may be required in these cases. Gastric decompression with a gastrostomy tube to minimize reflux and enteral feedings through a jejunostomy tube may permit healing of the rupture, provided the mediastinal sepsis is controlled.

CLINICAL POINTS TO REMEMBER

1. Boerhaave's syndrome is a thoracic surgical emergency.
2. Early recognition of the symptom complex and typical presentation of patients with Boerhaave's syndrome minimizes morbidity and mortality of patients with this disorder.
3. If primary closure is possible, a follow-up barium swallow is performed 7–10 days postoperatively and oral feeding reinstituted if no leak is evident.
4. Stricturing after repair may require intermittent dilations.

SELECTED READINGS

Derbes VJ, Mitchell RE Jr. The first translation (from original Latin, 1724) of the classic case report of rupture of the esophagus, with annotations (Hermann Boerhaave's "Atrocis, nec Descripti Prius, Morbi Historia"). Bull Med Libr Assoc 1955;43:217–219.

Postlethwait RW. Surgery of the Esophagus (2nd ed). Norwalk, CT: Appleton-Century-Crofts, 1986;161–189.

Sakamoto Y, Tanaka N, Furuya T, et al. Surgical management of late esophageal perforation. Thorac Cardiovasc Surg 1997;45:269–272.

4

Loss of Vision in a Man Carrying Groceries on Ice

John is returning from the grocery store with his weekly supply of food on a cold February evening. He lives alone. It is snowing lightly. Snow that melted earlier in the week when the weather was milder has refrozen into a layer of ice. Walking is difficult because of the light dusting of snow on the ice. John is holding two bags of groceries between his arms. He slips on the ice; both legs go out from beneath him, and he lands flat on his back. His large hat softens the blow to his occiput. He manages to pick himself up. He has a sharp pain on the right side of his chest but is not short of breath. He finds his house keys, opens his front door, and turns on the light. He thinks that the light must have burned out because it is still dark in the house; when he looks around, he realizes that he cannot see well, and, in fact, at this point cannot see at all. He feels around the living room for the phone and calls 911. He notices that his voice has changed quality and he sounds a bit like Donald Duck. He explains that he has fallen and now has lost his vision. The ambulance arrives and finds John as he appears in Figure 4-1.

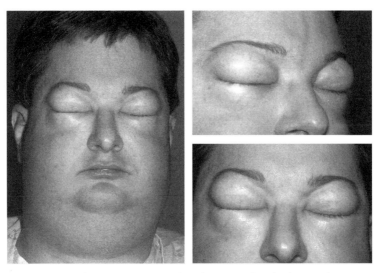

Figure 4-1 John's appearance when he arrived at the hospital.

DISCUSSION

Subcutaneous emphysema, or *surgical emphysema*, as it is called when it is associated with a thoracic surgical procedure, results in the tracking of air along the subcutaneous tissue planes. In John's case, a small rib fracture occurred when he fell on his back, and air from the torn lung quickly tracked along the mediastinal tissues, out of the thoracic outlet, and into the neck, and spread to the face and the tissues of the eyelids. The eyelids were nearly swollen shut under the pressure of the air, resulting in a perceived central vision loss. Air tracking around the larynx and pharynx caused the characteristic change in John's voice. Surgical emphysema can occur extremely quickly, depending on the volume of the air leak from the lung and the laxity of the tissue planes. Pneumothorax does not necessarily accompany these changes, but is a possibility.

Spontaneous pneumomediastinum can occur in asthmatics or in patients with pulmonary bullous disease. Air in the mediastinum can result in a classic Hamman's crunch (the sound of cardiac pulsations against the air) on auscultation. Palpable air in the tissues of the neck feels similar to the bubbles in packing crate material. Air can track down to the hands and the groin. When pneumomediastinum appears in patients who have had chest surgery, it is often caused by a chest tube that has kinked or plugged; air from the lung follows the chest tube and leaks around the subcutaneous tissues. Retaping the chest tube or placing the tube on suction is usually all that is required.

Generally, no treatment is required for pneumomediastinum, and reassurance of the patient and family is all that is needed. Subcutaneous placement of drains has been advocated; however, if streptococcus or staphylococcus is thereby introduced into the freshly expanded tissue planes, serious cellulitis can result. Sustained pressure on the eyelids displaces some of the air forcing them closed and "miraculously" re-establishes vision. On rare occasions, air can track into the pericardial sac and result in tension pneumopericardium that requires needle aspiration for hemodynamic compromise. Circumferential chest wall involvement that interferes with ventilation can occasionally indicate a need to place subcutaneous drains.

Pharyngeal, esophageal, and other gastrointestinal tract perforations are the most serious causes of air in the neck or mediastinum and require urgent evaluation. Gastrografin or barium evaluation of the gastrointestinal tract is required if the history suggests a gastrointestinal source for the air. Unrecognized gastrointestinal perforation can result in mediastinitis, neck fasciitis, peritonitis, and overwhelming sepsis and death.

CLINICAL POINTS TO REMEMBER

1. Subcutaneous emphysema, or surgical emphysema, results in the tracking of air along the subcutaneous tissue planes.
2. Air in the mediastinum can result in a classic Hamman's crunch on auscultation, which is the sound of the cardiac pulsations against the trapped air.
3. Generally, no treatment is required and reassurance of the patient and family is all that is needed.

SELECTED READINGS

Hampton SM, Cinnamond MJ. Subcutaneous emphysema as a complication of tonsillectomy. J Laryngol Otol 1997;111:1077–1078.

Kramer NR, Fine MD, McRae RG, Millman RP. Unusual complication of nasal CPAP: subcutaneous emphysema following facial trauma. Sleep 1997;20:895–897.

Saab M, Birkinshaw R. Blunt laryngeal trauma: an unusual case. Int J Clin Pract 1997;51:527.

5

Respiratory Arrest in an Old Man with Bad Breath

Grandpa Smith is a 78-year-old man whose grandchildren always kid him about his bad breath when they are instructed by their mother to give Grandpa a good-night kiss. His teeth were removed more than 10 years ago, but his dentures appear to fit well, and he religiously cleans them every night. Grandpa had read an article that outlined several causes of halitosis, including dental caries, gingivitis, and a bacterium that grows on the tongue, for which brushing the back of the tongue two to three times per day is recommended. He purchased the tongue brush, but it does not seem to help. He has noted some dysphagia over the past year and a peculiar gurgling sound in his neck while he is eating. He has also noticed that he can regurgitate undigested pieces of food into the back of his throat several hours after eating. He jokes with his daughter that he had developed an extra stomach, just like the old cows on the farm. He has lost some weight over the past 6 months and was hospitalized in the fall for right lower lobe pneumonia.

One Sunday, Grandpa Smith's daughter comes over and cooks a large roast with potatoes for dinner. Grandpa enjoys the meal and lies down on the couch for a nap afterwards. One hour later, while cleaning up the dishes, his daughter hears him coughing violently; she goes into the living room and finds him cyanotic and unconscious on the floor. She immediately starts cardiopulmonary resuscitation (CPR) but is unable to obtain an airway. She sweeps her finger around the back of his throat after removing his dentures, and is surprised to find a large piece of undigested meat lodged in his posterior pharynx. She is now able to establish an airway and, with jaw thrust and a few seconds of mouth-to-mouth resuscitation, he quickly regains consciousness. The emergency medical service is activated by calling 911, and Grandpa Smith is transported to the local ED with a patent airway and a stable blood pressure.

The story is related to the emergency physician. Grandpa Smith is admitted to the ICU, where he remains for 24 hours. He makes a full recovery. As part of his in-hospital workup, a barium swallow is obtained and found to be grossly abnormal, a finding thought to be compatible with a Zenker's diverticulum. An operation is performed.

DISCUSSION

A Zenker's diverticulum is a relatively uncommon abnormality of the junction of the pharynx and esophagus. It is a pulsion diverticulum that can grow to significant size, sometimes with minimal symptoms, although even individuals with smaller diverticula note some oropharyngeal dysphagia and food regurgitation. The primary cause is thought to be incomplete relaxation of the cricopharyngeal muscle when the inferior constrictor muscles of the pharynx constrict during swallowing.

Symptoms of a Zenker's diverticulum are often related to retained food in the diverticulum that can result in severe halitosis (as in Grandpa Smith's case); dysphagia, as the diverticulum expands; and respiratory symptoms that can range from a cough caused by the aspiration of liquid or solid contents of the sac to occlusion of the airway by dislodged food pieces. In Grandpa Smith's case, an upper airway obstruction was caused by a dislodged food piece.

A modified barium swallow with special attention to the swallowing mechanism usually demonstrates a midline protrusion at the level of the posterior hypopharyngeal wall, above the cricopharyngeus, and deviation to the patient's left side. A Zenker's diverticulum can vary in size from less than 1 cm to more than 10 cm. Rigid endoscopic evaluation should not be performed, because it can result in perforation of the thin-walled diverticulum. Flexible endoscopy should be used if there is a concern for an associated malignancy of the esophagus; such malignancies occur, but they are rare. Although some authors have studied the swallowing mechanisms and musculature of the area in great detail, motility studies are difficult to carry out in this region of the pharynx and esophagus.

In symptomatic patients, the diverticulum is surgically approached on the left side of the neck, medial to the carotid vessels. Care is taken not to injure the recurrent laryngeal nerve as it courses along the tracheo-esophageal groove. The diverticulum is usually resected, although some surgeons simply plexy the sac to the posterior pharyngeal musculature. If resection is performed, a stapling device or interrupted sutures at the neck of the sac are used. Closure is performed over a bougie to ensure that no narrowing of the esophagus or pharynx results. The cricopharyngeal muscle is completely divided, and the myotomy is often continued 3–4 cm along the cervical esophagus and 2–3 cm along the hypopharynx. A neck drain is placed, and feeding is started the next day.

Other diverticula in the esophagus can occur. Pulsion diverticula of the esophagus can appear distally, just proximal to the esophagogastric junction, and have a similar cause: a lack of coordination between relaxation of the lower esophageal sphincter and the contractions of the esophageal pressure waves. Traction diverticula occur in the midesophagus around the carina and are related to granulomatous disease, including tuberculosis and histoplasmosis. Often these diverticula do not cause symptoms and do not require surgery.

CLINICAL POINTS TO REMEMBER

1. A Zenker's diverticulum is a relatively uncommon abnormality of the junction of the pharynx and esophagus.
2. Respiratory arrest may be the initial presentation of Zenker's diverticula.
3. Rigid endoscopic evaluation should not be performed, because it can result in perforation of the thin-walled diverticulum.
4. In symptomatic patients, the diverticulum is surgically approached on the left side of the neck, medial to the carotid vessels.

SELECTED READINGS

Achkar E. Zenker's diverticulum. Dig Dis 1998; 16:144–151.

Gregoire J, Duranceau A. Surgical management of Zenker's diverticulum. Hepatogastroenterology 1992;39:132–138.

Ochando Cerdàn F, Moreno Gonzalez E, Hernandez Garcia D, et al. Diagnostic and treatment of Zenker's diverticulum: review of our series pharyngo-esophageal diverticula. Hepatogastroenterology 1998;45:447–450.

6

The Long-Forgotten Ride in a Small Car with a Large Friend

Bill works as a computer programmer for a software company in Silicon Valley. Over the past 2 weeks, he has noticed progressive shortness of breath on exertion. He has also noticed vague abdominal discomfort after meals and has avoided carbonated drinks for at least a month because he feels bloated and unable to belch after getting his usual caffeine fix from soft drinks. He has lost 10 lb over the past 3 months and experienced a loss of appetite that is unusual for him. This morning after breakfast, he was so short of breath after climbing a flight of stairs that his wife insisted he be evaluated in the local ED.

On arriving at the hospital, Bill is comfortable at rest but has dullness to percussion in the left lung base and distant breath sounds. A chest radiograph demonstrates a large hydropneumothorax involving the left hemithorax with little pulmonary parenchyma visible. The surgical resident is consulted and diagnoses Bill with a large pleural effusion that may, considering his history of vague gastrointestinal symptoms, anorexia, and progressive weight loss, represent a stage IV malignancy. Preparations are made for placing a chest tube to relieve symptoms and obtain a cytologic diagnosis.

The patient is positioned with his left chest elevated on a roll. His chest is prepared with 1% lidocaine, a skin wheal is raised, and a track into the fifth intercostal space in the midaxillary line is created using a 22-gauge needle. The needle is advanced into the chest and pleura with free return of fluid. A skin incision is made, and blunt dissection into the chest with a hemostat is performed. The pleura is punctured with the hemostat; it is expected that a large volume of pleural fluid will leak out, but none does. A slight sucking sound seems to confirm entrance into the pleura cavity.

Digital dissection of the chest reveals a soft structure that appears to be fluid filled but separate from the chest wall. Although soft, it does not move with respiration and does not feel like pulmonary tissue. Digital exploration to locate a possible loculated effusion is unsuccessful. The procedure is aborted at this time, and the skin incision is closed with an interrupted silk suture.

The surgical resident considers his procedural findings. He questions the patient closely about previous hospitalizations. Bill initially denies any previous medical illnesses, surgical procedures, or hospitalizations but then remembers an overnight stay in the ED of a small hospital in Oregon more than 6 months ago. He had spent a weekend at a high school reunion with a group of his friends and was involved in a motor vehicle accident. They were coming back from a party; the driver lost control of the car and went off the road into a ditch. Bill was sitting in the back seat of the small car, next to a high school buddy who was a lineman on the football team. He rolled sideways and hit Bill in the abdomen. No one appeared to have been injured in the accident, but the paramedics insisted that everyone involved be checked out in the local hospital. Chest radiographs, blood work, and physical examinations were unremarkable at that time, and, after 6 hours of observation, they were all released to enjoy the rest of the weekend.

On hearing this story, the surgical resident asks the nurse for an 18-Fr nasogastric tube. This is passed through Bill's nose and seems to go down the esophagus without difficulty, but it meets with some resistance at the level of the gastroesophageal junction. Immediately after the tube passes this area of slight resistance, more than 2 liters of gastric contents is aspirated. A second chest radiograph taken in the ED demonstrates an acute angulation of the nasogastric tube from the gastroesophageal junction into the apex of the left hemithorax. A diagnosis of delayed traumatic rupture of the left hemidiaphragm is made. The patient is admitted, hydrated, and prepared for elective surgery the next morning.

DISCUSSION

The diaphragm is a large, thin muscle that is arranged in an inverted J coursing from the sternum and fourth and fifth ribs anteriorly and extending to the L2 vertebrae posteriorly with insertion into the chest wall laterally. The muscle fibers connect to a large central tendon that flattens with shortening of the muscle fibers and acutely increases the volume of each hemithorax, decreasing the intrathoracic pressure and permitting the net movement of air from atmospheric pressure into the chest.

The diaphragm can be injured through both sharp and blunt traumas. Sharp injuries are more easily recognized and are usually related to knife or gunshot injuries, with both hemidiaphragms equally involved. Structures close to the diaphragm may be injured, including the liver and lung on the right and the stomach, spleen, splenic flexure of the colon, and lung on the left, depending on the level of the entrance and exit wounds. Posteriorly, the kidneys and retroperitoneal structures such as the aorta can be injured. The abdomen is explored first with chest tube monitoring of intrathoracic hemorrhage. Most sharp injuries to the diaphragm can be primarily closed without the need for prosthetic meshes. Shotgun or blast injuries that result in large tissue defects may require reconstruction with Gore-Tex mesh, either immediately after the initial injury or after some delay if extensive contamination of the operative field exists.

Blunt injuries usually result from a large increase in the intra-abdominal pressure with tearing of the central tendon in its posterior and lateral portions. Fewer blunt ruptures of the left hemidiaphragm occur than of the right hemidiaphragm (25% vs. 75%) because of the buttressing effect of the liver as it overlies the left hemidiaphragm. If the injury is recognized at the time of the initial accident, repair is performed by an abdominal approach with primary closure of the diaphragm and repositioning of the herniated abdominal organs in their proper anatomic locations (unlike type III or IV paraesophageal hernias, in which the mechanism of herniation is different and is associated with the development of a hernial sac. When diagnosis is delayed, a transthoracic approach is advisable, because multiple adhesions can form in the chest and make an abdominal approach more difficult.

Bill's symptoms over the 6 months after the accident are related to the progressive migration of the stomach through the defect, with resulting anorexia, vague abdominal discomfort, and inability to belch caused by acute angulation of the gastroesophageal junction as the stomach is drawn into the chest. The radiologist must be wary in diagnosing a hydropneumothorax, because the herniated stomach can slowly enlarge to fill virtually the entire hemithorax. In Bill's case, surgical exploration through the seventh intercostal space demonstrated not only the herniated stomach within the chest but also the spleen and a portion of the transverse colon. Fortunately, the surgical resident had adhered to the cardinal rule of digitally examining the chest before placing a chest tube. If a trocar chest tube had been used or dissection with the hemostat been more forceful, an iatrogenic gastrostomy or injury to the spleen or colon would have resulted, with disastrous consequences. Once the abdominal contents had been reduced, the defect in the diaphragm was primarily closed with nonabsorbable sutures, and the left lung, which had become progressively more compressed over the past several months, expanded nicely. The patient was discharged from the hospital 5 days later, having regained his appetite and love of carbonated drinks with significantly improved exercise performance.

CLINICAL POINTS TO REMEMBER

1. The diaphragm can be injured through both sharp and blunt mechanisms of trauma.
2. Sharp injuries are more easily recognized and are usually related to knife or gunshot injuries, with both hemidiaphragms equally involved.
3. Blunt injuries usually are caused by a large increase in the intra-abdominal

pressure with tearing of the central tendon in its posterior and lateral portions.
4. Clinicians must be wary in diagnosing a hydropneumothorax, because the herniated stomach can slowly enlarge to fill virtually the entire hemithorax.

SELECTED READING

Lucas C, Ledgerwood AM. Diaphragmatic Injury. In J Cameron (ed), Current Surgical Therapy (6th ed). St. Louis: Mosby, 1998;944–947.

7

A Marathon Runner with Shortness of Breath

Lynn is a 42-year-old businesswoman who frequently partici-
pates in local marathons. She is healthy and enjoys jogging
every day. On the day of the most important marathon in town,
Lynn is brought to the ED after collapsing on the twentieth
mile. According to her friends, she was feeling short of breath
and collapsed suddenly. Once awake, she insists on continuing
to run and finishing the marathon, but she collapses again. The
emergency medical system is called, and she is transported to
the hospital.

On arriving at the ED, she is unable to give an adequate history because of her altered mental status. According to a friend,
she had been drinking a lot of fluids before and during the race.
In addition, she was taking nonsteroidal anti-inflammatory
drugs (NSAIDs) for muscle pain relief. Physical examination
reveals an ill-appearing woman with evident respiratory distress. Her blood pressure is 110/80 mm Hg, her heart rate is 95
bpm, her temperature is 38.5°C, and her respiratory rate is 26
breaths per minute.

Lynn is lethargic but arousable. She has diminished breath
sounds bilaterally, but otherwise her physical examination is
unremarkable. Arterial blood gases reveal pH of 7.38, P_{CO_2} of
40 mm Hg, and P_{O_2} of 50 mm Hg. Chest radiography reveals
very discrete bilateral fluffy infiltrates with a normal cardiovascular silhouette (Figure 7-1). Serum electrolytes reveal sodium
of 118 mmol/liter, potassium of 4.5 mmol/liter, chloride of 98
mmol/liter, carbon dioxide of 22 mmol/liter, blood urea nitrogen of 22 mg/dl, and creatinine of 1 mg/dl. Lynn's mental status is rapidly deteriorating, and she is promptly intubated. Her
postintubation chest radiograph reveals worsening pulmonary
infiltrates (Figure 7-2). An immediate CT scan of the head
reveals diffuse cerebral edema.

She is admitted to the ICU and treated with 3% saline.
Within 24 hours of admission, her level of consciousness has
markedly improved. A repeat chest radiograph (Figure 7-3) is

completely clear after 2 days. She is extubated on the third day and has a favorable neurologic outcome. On follow-up at 6 months, the patient was neurologically intact, a magnetic resonance image of the brain was normal, and she was running again.

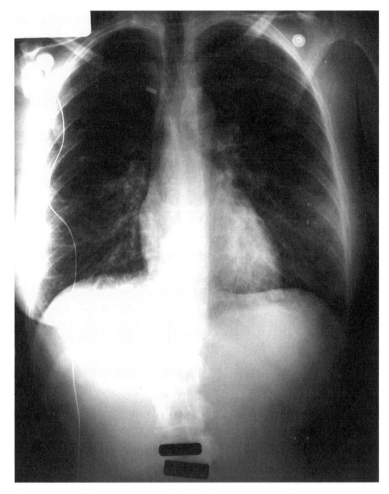

Figure 7-1 Chest x-ray on arrival at the emergency department.

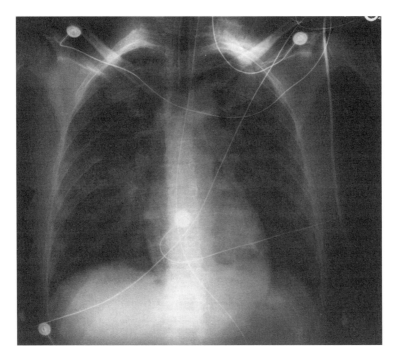

Figure 7-2   Chest x-ray immediately after intubation.

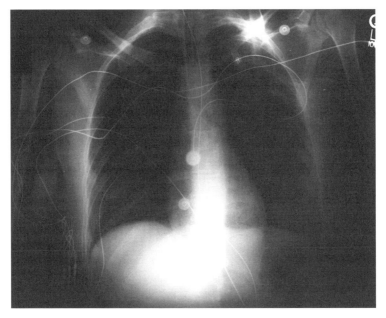

Figure 7-3   Chest x-ray after treatment with 3% saline.

DISCUSSION

This patient's history of overexertion and increased water intake, as well as of use of NSAIDs (which impair the ability of the kidney to excrete water), suggests a diagnosis of hyponatremic encephalopathy. Serum electrolytes showed hyponatremia (118 mmol/liter), and serum osmolality was low in this patient, confirming the clinical diagnosis. A CT scan of the head revealed generalized brain edema. The development of an initial presentation of hyponatremic encephalopathy from respiratory insufficiency (noncardiogenic pulmonary edema), however, is most noteworthy. This syndrome has been described in detail and can produce noncardiogenic pulmonary edema and hypercapnic respiratory failure.

Hyponatremia (serum sodium of ≤135 mmol/liter) is the most common electrolyte abnormality found in hospitalized patients. Because patients with many types of serious illnesses, such as congestive heart failure, cirrhosis of the liver, nephrosis, acquired immunodeficiency syndrome, tuberculosis, head injury, malignancy, and gastrointestinal illnesses, often have associated hyponatremia, separating the morbidity and mortality that result from the underlying medical condition from morbidity and mortality caused by hyponatremia can be difficult.

Since the 1980s, numerous studies have shown that significant morbidity and mortality are associated with symptomatic hyponatremia that is unrelated to any underlying medical conditions. Children (because of physical factors) and women of childbearing age (through hormonally mediated mechanisms) are especially susceptible to brain damage or death from symptomatic hyponatremia. This catastrophe may occur in both children and young women at levels of serum sodium as high as 133 mmol/liter, a level which is usually asymptomatic in men.

Acute hyponatremia can cause brain swelling when water moves from plasma to the brain in order to lower brain osmolality so that it matches hypotonic plasma osmolality. When the increase in brain volume exceeds 5–7% of its normal volume, death can result from increased intracranial pressure and subsequent brain swelling and herniation through the foramen magnum. Hyponatremic brain edema is normally prevented by the transport of osmotically active solutes out of brain cells by processes that involve the Na^+/K^+-ATPase pump, amino acids, and potassium and calcium channels. The susceptibility of premenopausal women to complications from symptomatic hyponatremia may result in part from impaired cerebral osmotic adaptation in women.

Patients with symptomatic hyponatremia may develop a symptom complex that includes opisthotonos, respiratory depression, impaired response to verbal and painful stimuli, bizarre behavior, fecal or urinary incontinence, visual or auditory hallucinations and lethargy. Patients with symptomatic hyponatremia may also develop respiratory arrest, dilated pupils, hypertension, and abnormal temperature regulation within 24 hours of onset. In all patients with symptomatic hyponatremia, the presenting symptoms are often dramatic (e.g., seizures or respiratory arrest) and may indicate an advanced process for which no therapy is likely to produce a good outcome.

Patients with symptomatic hyponatremia (serum sodium of ≤128 mmol/liter) should be treated with hypertonic sodium chloride (514 mmol/liter) using an infusion pump, with the infusion designed to raise plasma sodium at a rate of approximately 1 mmol/liter per hour until the patient becomes alert and seizure-free, the plasma sodium has increased by 20–25 mmol/liter, or a serum sodium of approximately 125–130 mmol/liter is achieved, whichever occurs first. At that time, hypertonic NaCl should be discontinued. The patient should be moved to a location where constant monitoring can be provided, such as the ICU. Monitoring of plasma electrolytes should be carried out every 2 hours during the initial period of correction until the patient becomes neurologically stable. In addition to hypertonic sodium chloride, therapy may include intubation and assisted mechanical ventilation when required. This regimen may require modification in patients with severe renal or cardiac disease. Because of the danger of brain damage, the serum sodium should never be acutely elevated to hypernatremic or normonatremic levels. In addition, because brain damage has also been associated with acute excessive changes in serum sodium, the serum sodium should not be elevated by more than 25 mmol/liter during the initial 48 hours of therapy.

CLINICAL POINTS TO REMEMBER

1. Symptomatic hyponatremia is especially likely to result in brain damage or death in children and women of childbearing age.
2. Noncardiogenic pulmonary edema and respiratory arrest can occur in patients with hyponatremia.
3. Patients with symptomatic hyponatremia (serum sodium of ≤128 mmol/liter) should be treated with hypertonic sodium chloride (514 mmol/liter).

SELECTED READINGS

Arieff AI. Hyponatremia, convulsions, respiratory arrest, and permanent brain damage after elective surgery in healthy women. N Engl J Med 1986;314:1529–1535.

Ayus JC, Arieff AI. Pulmonary complications of hyponatremic encephalopathy. Noncardiogenic pulmonary edema and hypercapnic respiratory failure. Chest 1995;107:517–521.

Ayus JC, Varon J, Fraser CL. Pathogenesis and management of hyponatremic encephalopathy. Curr Opin Crit Care 1995;1:452–459.

Ayus JC, Wheeler JM, Arieff AI. Postoperative hyponatremic encephalopathy in menstruant women. Ann Intern Med 1992;117:891–897.

8

The Cancer Patient with a Large Left-Sided Pleural Effusion and the Intensive Care Unit Resident with Stubby Fingers

Mrs. Smith is a 48-year-old, moderately obese housewife who was diagnosed with a malignant fibrous histiocytoma in her right leg 4 years ago. She was treated with high-dose ifosfamide and Adriamycin followed by local excision of the primary tumor and radiation therapy, and she was able to maintain function in her leg. Mrs. Smith developed Adriamycin-induced cardiomyopathy with an estimated ejection fraction of 25%. She was reasonably functional while maintained on digoxin.

Mrs. Smith was doing well until recently, when she experienced increasing shortness of breath with exertion. She thinks this may be related to worsening of her cardiomyopathy but is found to have diminished breath sounds in her left chest with dullness to percussion. A chest radiograph confirms the presence of a large left-sided pleural effusion that layers during left lateral decubitus positioning. This is tapped through the posterior eighth intercostal space and found to be bloody. Cytologic assessment confirms metastatic disease. Two liters of fluid is aspirated, and her respiratory status immediately improves. A chest radiograph shows full expansion of the left lung.

A CT scan shows multiple small lesions within the pulmonary parenchyma consistent with miliary metastatic spread. Possible treatment options for her case are discussed at a multidisciplinary planning conference. Over the next 24 hours, she again deteriorates from a respiratory point of view; she requires admission to the medical ICU and is placed on supplemental oxygen (80% mask).

Another chest radiograph shows silhouetting of the left hemidiaphragm and cardiac border and a pleural effusion occupying at least 50% of the left hemithorax. The thoracic resident is asked to place a chest tube for symptomatic relief and subsequent talc sclerosis when the drainage has subsided and the lung is re-expanded.

Stubby-fingered Dr. John Snowden is the resident on call that evening. He reviews the radiographs and obtains consent from the patient. A roll is placed behind her back to rotate her left side anteriorly. She is connected to an oxygen saturation monitor and an automatic blood pressure cuff. Midazolam is administered intravenously. A wide chest prep with povidone is performed, and 1% lidocaine is infiltrated into the seventh intercostal space in what is felt to be the midaxillary line. A spinal needle is required, because of the patient's obesity, to anesthetize the intercostal space. A bloody pleural effusion is aspirated. A 2-cm skin incision is made, the subcutaneous tissues and chest wall musculature are spread with a hemostat down to the interspace, and the interspace is entered. Immediately, a large amount of bloody effusion comes out. An attempt is made to digitally palpate the lung to ensure that no adhesions are present, but the resident cannot get his finger into the chest.

Dr. Snowden decides to guide the chest tube posteriorly, using the trocar supplied with the chest tube. The tube is advanced. A slight resistance is encountered. He pushes slightly with the trocar to force the chest tube through what he thinks is the intercostal space. Immediately, the chest tube fills with a bloody fluid that he interprets as the bloody pleural effusion. As he withdraws the trocar to advance the chest tube, the fluid in the chest tube squirts across the room. It is evident that the fluid in the tube is frank blood under arterial pressure. Left ventricular insertion is suspected.

DISCUSSION

This case illustrates several important points. Any patient with a history of cardiac failure, cardiomyopathy, or ventricular dilation must be approached with caution before placement of any percutaneous tubes or needles. When cardiac enlargement is present, the left ventricle will move laterally and inferiorly. Rolling the patient may fool the physician into thinking the patient is more lateral than he or she really is.

Whenever a chest tube is inserted into a hemithorax, it is imperative that the intrathoracic structures be palpated to ensure that no adherence of the lung is present, that the heart is proximate, and that supradiaphragmatic placement will avoid injury to the spleen, stomach, and colon on the left and the liver on the right. If a surgeon's finger is too short to feel the intrathoracic structures, the skin incision must be increased. A trocar catheter should *never* be used. If a metal trocar is used to guide a chest tube posteriorly, it must be retracted so that no injury to an intrathoracic structure can occur. A dilated left ventricle, which may rest just below the intercostal space, can be easily injured by a hemostat or chest tube trocar. If a chest tube is inserted into a cardiac chamber or other vascular structure, it should be clamped rather than removed, and the patient should be transported immediately to the operating room for emergency thoracotomy and controlled removal. In this case, a felt-pledgetted mattress suture was placed around the chest tube, the chest tube was removed, and the left ventricular apex was repaired with a single stitch.

CLINICAL POINTS TO REMEMBER

1. Whenever a chest tube is inserted into a hemithorax, it is imperative that the intrathoracic structures be palpated.
2. A trocar catheter should *never* be used when placing a chest tube.
3. If a chest tube is inserted into a cardiac chamber or other vascular structure, it should be clamped rather than removed, and the patient should be transported immediately to the operating room for emergency thoracotomy and controlled removal.

SELECTED READINGS

Chan L, Reilly KM, Henderson C, et al. Complication rates of tube thoracostomy. Am J Emerg Med 1997;15:368–370.

Deakin CD. Morbidity in 624 patients requiring prehospital chest tube decompression. J Trauma 1998;44:1115–1117.

Iberti TJ, Stern PM. Chest tube thoracostomy. Crit Care Clin 1992;8:879–895.

Quigley RL. Thoracentesis and chest tube drainage. Crit Care Clin 1995;11:111–126.

Tomlinson MA, Treasure T. Insertion of a chest drain: how to do it. Br J Hosp Med 1997;58: 248–252.

9

A Kid with a Cough After a Christmas Party

Michael, a 3-year-old boy, goes to his grandparents' home for a Christmas party. During this event, presents are exchanged, and Michael receives his first construction set. He is very excited and immediately wants to play with it. He goes into a room with his cousin Darryl (age 4). While their parents are looking for them, the children fight forcefully with each other over who will play with the construction set. A few minutes later, Darryl comes out of the room screaming that Michael will not let him play with his toy and that they had a fight.

The next morning, Michael has several episodes of nonproductive cough. His mother calls his primary care provider, who prescribes a cough suppressant and rest. Over the next few days, Michael continues to cough and is seen by his pediatrician, who diagnoses him with a respiratory infection and prescribes an oral antibiotic for 10 days. After Michael has completed his antibiotic course, he continues to have nonproductive cough and develops fever and chills. His mother takes him to the local ED.

On arrival at the ED, Michael appears quite ill. He is tachypneic and tachycardic with a rectal temperature of 39°C. Physical examination reveals a young child in acute distress with markedly diminished breath sounds at the right lower lobe area. A posteroanterior chest radiograph is obtained and reveals the presence of a foreign body with partial collapse of the right lower lobe (Figure 9-1).

Michael is taken to the operating room for an emergency bronchoscopy. During the procedure, a 1-in. nail is retrieved from his right bronchus intermedius. The remainder of the tracheobronchial tree shows no evidence of endobronchial lesions or foreign bodies. He is treated with IV antibiotics for 2 days and discharged home with significant improvement in his symptomatology. On follow-up 6 weeks later, Michael is asymptomatic and is still playing with his construction set (though only under parental supervision).

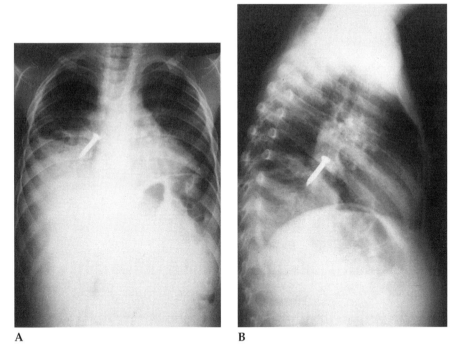

A   B

Figure 9-1   These posteroanterior **(A)** and lateral **(B)** chest radiographs were obtained in the emergency department.

DISCUSSION

This case is a slightly atypical foreign body aspiration. The radiographic findings are striking and allow the clinician to "nail" the diagnosis. Foreign body aspiration is a relatively common event among children. Nuts have been described as the most frequent offenders, and most aspirations occur in young children, with 95% of aspirations occurring in children younger than 10 years. The majority of patients present with symptoms more than 24 hours after aspiration. A clear history of aspiration is commonly lacking.

The symptoms of foreign body aspiration vary according to the site and degree of obstruction. Foreign bodies located in the intrathoracic trachea or bronchi tend to produce wheezing, whereas extrathoracic obstructions lead to inspiratory stridor. Radiographic evaluation should be performed, and both inspiratory and expiratory films should be considered. The clinician must remember that many foreign bodies are not radio-opaque.

Pneumonia distal to the obstructed bronchus may result in fever, sputum production, and bronchiectasis if the foreign object is not removed. Removal of many foreign bodies in the tracheobronchial tree may require rigid bronchoscopy performed by a skilled operator. Occasionally bronchoscopic extraction is not possible and a surgical resection is necessary.

CLINICAL POINTS TO REMEMBER

1. Aspiration of foreign objects is common among children under the age of 10, with most occurring in children between the ages of 1 and 3 years.
2. Many foreign bodies are not radiographically visible, and failure to see a foreign body on chest radiograph does not exclude this diagnosis.
3. Retained foreign bodies ultimately lead to recurrent bouts of pneumonia secondary to airway obstruction.

SELECTED READINGS

Mansour Y, Beck R, Danino J, Bentur L. Resolution of severe bronchiectasis after removal of long-standing retained foreign body. Pediatr Pulmonol 1998;25:130–132.

Messner AH. Pitfalls in the diagnosis of aerodigestive tract foreign bodies. Clin Pediatr 1998;37: 359–365.

10

I'm OK⁺,
You're Not OK⁺

Wolfgang is a 67-year-old gentleman with a history of diabetes and hypertension who is admitted to the hospital on a Thursday night with abdominal pain and fever. His physical examination is initially unremarkable, except for midepigastric pain and a battery of screening laboratory studies revealing mild leukocytosis, and did not suggest a specific diagnosis. Because of Wolfgang's continued discomfort and a desire not to mask significant intra-abdominal pathology, Dr. Z, intern on call, prescribed ketorolac, 60 mg IV every 6 hours around the clock. After 2 hours, Dr. Z receives a call from the laboratory about abnormal lab results. Wolfgang has an amylase of 1,024 IU and a lipase of 17,890 IU. Mild dyspnea is also noted, and Dr. Z places a nasogastric tube to decompress his abdomen and improve his shortness of breath.

Six hours after admission, Wolfgang has become lethargic and acutely dyspneic and nearly goes into respiratory arrest. He is immediately transferred to the ICU, where he is mechanically ventilated, central venous access is obtained, and total parenteral alimentation is instituted while the previously ordered therapy continues.

Over the weekend, Wolfgang has some improvement in pulmonary function. Extubation is planned for early Monday morning. At 11:30 PM on Sunday, the ICU nurse in charge of Wolfgang tells the intern on call, Dr. Y, that the patient has developed a change in his respiratory rhythm. Dr. Y orders an electrocardiogram (ECG) and leaves for the ICU immediately. On arrival at the ICU, Dr. Y reviews Wolfgang's ECG (Figure 10-1). Being more astute than Dr. Z, Dr. Y interprets the ECG as reflecting hyperkalemia and rapidly administers calcium, bicarbonate, glucose, and insulin and gives Wolfgang two doses of nebulized albuterol (0.25 mg in 2 cc of NS). A second ECG is shown in Figure 10-2.

Electrolytes drawn at the time of the initial ECG subsequently reveal serum potassium of 8 mmol/liter and creatinine of 5 mg/dl. Although nonoliguric, Wolfgang's renal function has rapidly deteriorated in the setting of his pancreatitis and the continued administration of an NSAID in a patient with a background of mild renal insufficiency.

After a protracted stay in the ICU, Wolfgang's pulmonary and renal function improve and he is able to be discharged from the hospital. Dr. Z learns a great lesson about the pitfalls of NSAIDs and the need for monitoring electrolytes, particularly in patients receiving total parenteral nutrition with potassium supplementation.

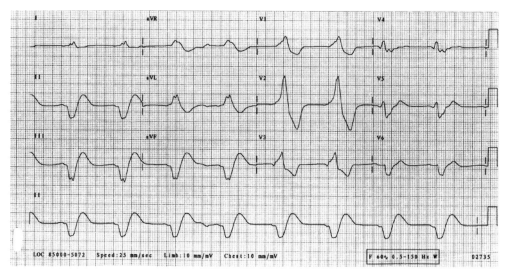

Figure 10-1 Wolfgang's initial electrocardiogram.

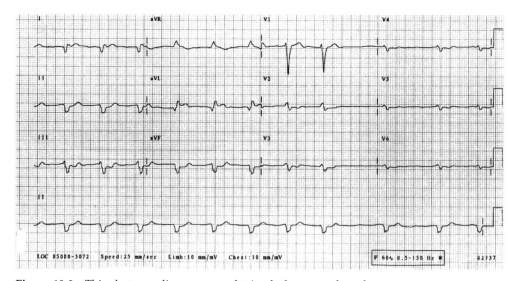

Figure 10-2 This electrocardiogram was obtained after secondary therapy.

DISCUSSION

Potassium [K$^+$] is the most abundant intracellular cation. Only approximately 2% of total body potassium is in the extracellular fluid. Intracellular potassium is responsible for maintaining cell volume and for resting membrane potential. A number of factors regulate potassium movement in and out of cells. Release of potassium from cells contributes to hyperkalemia in acidosis, poorly controlled diabetes mellitus, beta blockade, hyperkalemic periodic paralysis, hyperosmolar states, and digitalis toxicity. Inadequate renal excretion occurs in patients with advanced renal failure, deficiencies of adrenal hormones, and numerous drugs. These include potassium-sparing diuretics, NSAIDs, angiotensin-converting enzyme inhibitors, and cyclosporine.

Severe hyperkalemia is a frequent finding in patients with massive in vivo hemolysis or tumor lysis syndrome. Potassium ingestion seldom results in hyperkalemia if renal function is normal, except when excessive parenteral potassium supplements have been administered. However, patients with renal insufficiency may develop severe hyperkalemia.

The principal clinical abnormalities of hyperkalemia are neuromuscular and cardiac in nature. Weakness, paresthesias, and paralysis can occur but are usually overshadowed by cardiac disturbances. These include progressive ECG appearance of peaked T waves, flattened P waves, prolonged PR interval, and widening of the QRS complex, the last of which is well demonstrated by Wolfgang's first ECG. The development of a sine-wave pattern presages the onset of ventricular fibrillation or asystole.

The treatment of hyperkalemia is outlined in Table 10-1. Calcium does not affect the serum potassium but rather antagonizes the cardiac toxicity of hyperkalemia. Glucose/insulin and bicarbonate infusions lower serum [K$^+$] by stimulating cellular potassium entry. Kayexalate is used to augment fecal potassium excretion; it is relatively ineffective unless the patient develops diarrhea or loose stools. Dialysis is an extremely effective treatment for life-threatening hyperkalemia. Diuretics and aldosterone analogues are occa-

Table 10-1 Therapy for hyperkalemia

Therapy	Onset of action
10% calcium gluconate, 10–30 ml IV	<5 mins
50% dextrose, 50 ml and regular insulin, 5 IU IV q30min	15–30 mins
NaHCO$_3$, 50 ml (50 mEq) IV q30min 4 times/day	15–30 mins
Kayexalate in sorbitol, 30–60 g PO or PR q4–6h	1–2 hrs
Dialysis	5–15 mins

sionally useful adjunctive measures. The use of beta-adrenergic agents (i.e., albuterol) via nebulizations has received considerable attention for the acute management of hyperkalemia: A reduction of approximately 1 mmol/liter is seen after their administration. Like the administration of insulin and glucose, beta-adrenergic administration results in the intracellular shift of potassium. This is a transient phenomenon that allows the institution of more definitive therapy.

CLINICAL POINTS TO REMEMBER

1. Potassium ingestion seldom results in hyperkalemia if renal function is normal, except when excessive parenteral potassium supplements have been administered.
2. The principal clinical abnormalities of hyperkalemia are neuromuscular and cardiac in nature.
3. Calcium does not affect the serum potassium but rather antagonizes the cardiac toxicity of hyperkalemia.
4. Dialysis is very effective for life-threatening hyperkalemia.

SELECTED READINGS

Brennan S, Lederer ED. Severe Electrolyte Disturbances. In JB Hall, GA Schmidt, LDH Wood (eds), Principles of Critical Care. New York: McGraw-Hill, 1992;1930–1945.

Kunis KL, Lowenstein J. The emergency treatment of hyperkalemia. Med Clin North Am 1981; 65:165–176.

11

The Kind Resident and the Dyspneic Patient

Phil is a 63-year-old diabetic man with a strong aversion to health care. When initially diagnosed with type II diabetes mellitus, he strongly resisted his physician's assertion that he had a significant illness. His compliance with his therapeutic regimen could best be described as casual. In the days leading up to Phil's admission to the hospital, he developed a cough that produced scant amounts of yellow sputum and a fever. He became increasingly thirsty and needed to urinate frequently. Although Phil's wife pleaded with him to seek medical attention, it was not until he became lethargic that an ambulance was called and he was transported to the ED of the local hospital.

Phil's initial evaluation in the ED reveals that he is acutely ill, with a room air oxygen saturation (Sa_{O_2}) of 80% and a finger-stick glucose of 500 mg/dl. He is immediately transported to the ICU for diagnosis and treatment of his present condition. Dr. Stick, medical intern in the ICU, evaluates Phil and finds that he is tachycardic to 140 bpm; hypotensive, with a blood pressure of 97/54 mm Hg; and has a respiratory rate of 33 breaths per minute. On supplemental oxygen, Phil's Sa_{O_2} improves to 92%. However, he is still dyspneic and complains fiercely when the nursing staff attempts to lay him flat.

IV access cannot be obtained peripherally, and Dr. Stick prepares for the insertion of a central venous line. Phil is prepared and draped, and, because of his complaints on being supine, he is allowed to remain in a slightly head-up position. Dr. Stick is able to cannulate the vessel with some difficulty, but while he is inserting the dilator, Phil's pulse oximeter begins to sound an alarm. Dr. Stick quickly inserts the central venous catheter and prepares for emergent intubation. Within minutes, Dr. Stick skillfully intubates Phil and listens for bilateral breath sounds—he is concerned that pneumothorax may be the cause of Phil's desaturation. A chest radiograph (Figure 11-1) reveals no pneumothorax, and Dr. Stick, confused about what has occurred, contacts the staff intensivist.

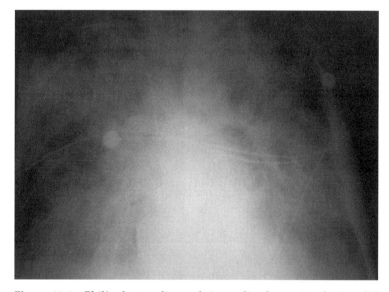

Figure 11-1 Phil's chest radiograph immediately postintubation did not reveal pneumothorax.

DISCUSSION

Placement of central venous catheters is an everyday occurrence in the modern ICU. The need for frequent blood sampling, administration of fluids and medications, and hemodynamic monitoring makes these devices an essential part of the management of some patients.

No absolute contraindications to central venous access exist. Relative contraindications may include bleeding diathesis and central venous thrombosis. The choice of central cannulation route depends on the clinical circumstances and the skill of the operator. Subclavian insertion has a higher risk of pneumothorax. It also presents a noncompressible vascular puncture site.

The following descriptions of approaches to central cannulation may be valuable to the reader.

Internal Jugular Catheterization

Informed consent should be obtained before internal jugular catheterization is attempted in the nonemergent setting. The physician should wash, gown, and glove; the operative site is gently prepared with iodophor solution and draped with sterile towels.

In an anterior approach to internal jugular catheterization, the patient is positioned in a 15- to 20-degree Trendelenburg position, and the headboard of the bed is removed. The internal jugular vein lies beneath the sternocleidomastoid muscle and slightly in front of the carotid artery. In the anterior approach, the carotid artery is palpated (with the left index and middle fingers), the puncture site is infiltrated with 1% lidocaine, and a finding needle is passed immediately lateral to the carotid pulsation, beneath the medial edge of the sternocleidomastoid muscle at the level of the thyroid cartilage. The needle is advanced at an angle of approximately 30 degrees to the skin (directed toward the ipsilateral nipple); the vessel should be encountered within 3 cm. When gentle suction on the syringe produces a rush of venous blood, the needle is removed and the procedure is repeated with a larger-gauge introducer needle on a 5- or 10-ml Luer-Lok syringe. Once the venous puncture has been achieved, a guidewire is passed into

the vessel (a vessel dilator can be used), and the venous catheter is inserted over the wire through a very small skin incision made over the wire. The wire subsequently is removed and intravenous extension tubing attached.

The middle approach to internal jugular catheterization is performed with the patient supine in a 20-degree Trendelenburg position and the patient's head slightly turned to the contralateral side. Local anesthetic is infiltrated at the junction of the sternal and clavicular heads of the sternocleidomastoid muscle. The needle is inserted at an angle of approximately 30 degrees to the skin and again directed toward the ipsilateral nipple. The vessel should be entered within 2–3 cm of insertion. Once vascular access has been obtained, the procedure is repeated with the introducer needle, the guidewire is passed through the needle, and cannulation is completed as above.

The posterior approach also begins with the patient positioned in a 20-degree Trendelenburg position and with the patient's head facing the contralateral shoulder. After the skin is prepared and local anesthetic administered, as in the anterior and middle approaches, the needle is inserted through the skin at the posterolateral margin of the sternocleidomastoid muscle (approximately 4 cm above the sternoclavicular junction). This is approximately the point at which the external jugular vein crosses the posterior margin of the sternocleidomastoid muscle, a commonly used landmark. The needle is advanced in a caudal and medial direction, aiming at the contralateral nipple. Once venous access with the introducer needle has been obtained, a guidewire is placed into the catheter and cannulation proceeds.

Subclavian Vein Cannulation

Before subclavian vein cannulation, the patient is prepared and positioned in a manner analogous to that for internal jugular vein cannulation. A rolled-up towel should be placed longitudinally between the scapulae to allow the shoulders to drop back. The patient's head is turned 45 degrees away from the side of intended placement. The puncture site is identified approximately 1 cm below the inferior margin of the clavicle at the junction of the medial and middle two-thirds. The region is infiltrated with 1% lidocaine, and lidocaine is also injected into the periosteum of the clavicle. The anesthetic needle is removed and the introducer needle inserted into the skin with the tip aimed at the suprasternal notch, passing just beneath the clavicle. The bevel of the needle should be pointed toward the head (cephalad). When free flow of blood is obtained from the introducer needle, the bevel can be rotated 180 degrees to facilitate thoracic placement of the guidewire. The catheter is threaded, the wire is removed, fluid flow is established, and the catheter is secured.

Femoral Vein

An approach to internal jugular catheterization through the femoral vein is easily performed in most patients. The patient is placed supine, knees extended, and the foot of the anticipated cannulation site is rotated outward 15–30 degrees. The site of insertion is cleaned and prepared as noted previously, and the region is draped.

The insertion point is identified; it lies 2–3 cm inferior to the inguinal ligament, 1–2 cm medial to the femoral pulse. (The reader is reminded of the *navl* mnemonic for the structures in this region: *n*erve, *a*rtery, *v*ein, *l*ymphatics.) A 22-gauge finder needle is commonly used to infiltrate a local anesthetic as well as to localize the vessel. After the femoral vein has been found, the introducer needle is placed on a syringe and inserted into the femoral vein. A flexible guidewire is placed, and the needle is exchanged for the vascular cannula; the catheter is then secured.

Complications

Complications of central venous access include infection, pneumothorax (more common with a subclavian approach), hemothorax, chylothorax, intrapleural infusion of IV fluids, dysrhythmias, thrombosis, pericardial tamponade, neurologic injuries, and hematomas.

Air embolism is a rarely recognized complication of central venous cannulation in critically ill patients. It occurs when air enters the vasculature and travels to the pulmonary cir-culation, causing respiratory embarrassment and frequently cardiovascular collapse. To develop, air embolism requires a pressure gradient that favors entry of air into the vessel. Although the air might be at atmospheric pressure, intravascular pressure may be subatmospheric. Any vein above the heart is likely to have subatmospheric intravascular pressure. The strong negative intrathoracic pressure generated in dyspneic patients like Phil, who demanded an upright posture during the attempted central venous cannulation, contributes to the development of the pressure gradient necessary for an air embolism.

The respiratory consequences of air embolism are substantial. Intravascular air is carried into the pulmonary vasculature, and the abnormal air-blood interface is thought to interact with plasma proteins, creating cellular debris, and with the activation of white blood cells, facilitating injury to the pulmonary capillaries. Alveolar flooding is caused by an increase in capillary permeability, as occurred in Phil's case (see Figure 11-1). Extrathoracic manifestations of air embolism may occur. Bubbles may pass to the left side of the heart via a patent foramen ovale and create peripheral embolization. A typical manifestation is ischemia in the brain, skin (*livedo reticularis*), and other organs.

Air embolism is usually recognized by acute hypoxemic respiratory failure occurring in a setting that predisposes to the condition. Once it has been recognized, prevention of further embolization is paramount. Standard treatment is similar to the treatment for any patient with acute respiratory distress syndrome: airway protection, assisted mechanical ventilation, and the use of supplemental oxygen and end-expiratory pressure as necessary.

It may be possible for a qualified physician in a cardiac catheterization laboratory to retrieve air from the venous circulation or the right heart. This should not be considered routine management, because significant amounts of air usually cannot be removed with cardiac catheterization with air bubble removal. Head-down, left lateral decubitus positioning of the patient has been recommended, but data proving the efficacy of this position are not available. Hyperbaric oxygen therapy theoretically should reduce bubble size. However, critically ill patients are seldom treated with this modality.

CLINICAL POINTS TO REMEMBER

1. Air embolism is a rarely recognized complication of central venous cannulation in critically ill patients.
2. Air embolism is usually recognized by acute hypoxemic respiratory failure.
3. The respiratory consequences of air embolism are substantial.
4. In some situations, it may be possible to retrieve air from the venous circulation or the right heart.

SELECTED READINGS

Fitchet A, Fitzpatrick AP. Central venous air embolism causing pulmonary oedema mimicking left ventricular failure. BMJ 1998;316:604–606.

Lam KK, Hutchinson RC, Gin T. Severe pulmonary oedema after venous air embolism. Can J Anaesth 1993;40:964–967.

Palmon SC, Moore LE, Lundberg J, Toung T. Venous air embolism: a review. J Clin Anesth 1997; 9:251–257.

Tibbles PM, Edelsberg JS. Hyperbaric oxygen therapy. N Engl J Med 1996;334:1642–1648.

Varon J, Fromm RE. Special Techniques. In J Varon (ed), Practical Guide to the Care of the Critically Ill Patient. St. Louis: Mosby–Year Book, 1994;321–339.

12

A Tall Man with Thick Glasses and Chest Pain

Bill, an active, athletic, 34-year-old man, experiences some chest discomfort while playing basketball. He goes in for a lay-up and notes an acute onset of chest discomfort that persists until his arrival at the hospital. Bill is alert and oriented; he has blood pressure of 110/80 mm Hg, heart rate of 60 bpm, and respiratory rate of 20 breaths per minute. He is a tall, thin, young-appearing man in moderate distress. His lungs are clear to auscultation and percussion, and the cardiac examination shows a normal jugular venous pressure, symmetric and strong carotid pulses, and normal heart sounds. An ECG is obtained 1 hour after the onset of symptoms and demonstrates sinus bradycardia at a rate of 56 bpm and normal axis and left ventricular hypertrophy by voltage criteria, with 2 mm of ST segment elevation in leads V_{1-3}.

Dr. H is on call and, given the history and the ECG changes, entertains a diagnosis of anteroseptal myocardial infarction. Because onset was acute, Bill is considered a candidate for thrombolytic therapy, and recombinant tissue plasminogen activator is administered.

Shortly after initiation of the thrombolytic therapy, Bill sits up abruptly, removes his thick glasses, and says, "I don't feel well" as he falls back to the bed. Repeat vital signs show a systolic pressure of 60 mm Hg. An echocardiogram is performed emergently and demonstrates a small pericardial effusion, concentric left ventricular hypertrophy, and normal left ventricular wall motion. Thrombolysis and heparin are discontinued, and fluids and IV catecholamines are begun. Despite this therapy, Bill remains hypotensive, with a systolic blood pressure of approximately 70 mm Hg. He is developing episodes of confusion and restlessness, and a repeat echocardiogram is performed, demonstrating an increase in the pericardial effusion with right ventricular diastolic collapse. He complains of worsening chest pain and of epigastric pain with a pleuritic component. The abdomen is distended, and complete disappearance of peripheral pulses with inspiration is noted.

Bill is transferred immediately to the cardiac catheterization laboratory, where right heart hemodynamics show elevation and equalization of diastolic pressures in the right atrium, pulmonary artery, and pulmonary occlusion pressures. On fluoroscopy, Bill's mediastinum appears widened, and a diagnosis of possible aortic dissection is entertained. An aortogram is obtained; it shows a type I aortic dissection with normal coronary arteries and mild aortic regurgitation. Bill is taken to emergency surgery for resection of the dissection and replacement with a graft by means of total cardiopulmonary bypass. Postoperatively, Bill develops acute respiratory distress syndrome, but he recovers and is discharged on the tenth postoperative day. He has now decided that lay-ups are out of his repertoire.

DISCUSSION

Chest pain is a common diagnosis for which patients are admitted to ICUs. A broad differential diagnosis, including many life-threatening illnesses, must be considered. Ischemic heart disease leads the list of concerns, but, as this case shows, other conditions may be present.

Bill's appearance was suggestive of Marfan syndrome, an inherited disorder that greatly increases the risk of aortic dissection. More than 2,000 new cases of aortic dissection occur each year in the United States. Approximately 75% of patients with dissections involving the ascending aorta die within 2 weeks if untreated. Prompt diagnosis and appropriate early intervention have led to dramatic improvements in outcome.

Aortic dissection was first documented in 1760, when King George II of England died while straining on the commode. At autopsy, he was found to have hematoma of the ascending aortic wall, an intimal tear, and blood in the pericardium. Although the prosector described this as a saccular aneurysm, the report is now considered to be the first description of aortic dissection. It was Morgagni, 1 year later, who first used the term *aortic dissection*, but it was not until 1856 that antemortem diagnosis was first accomplished, by Swaine and Latham.

The first attempted surgical repair of an aortic dissection was performed in 1935. Mortality remained high until DeBakey, Cooley, and Creech performed the first successful repair in 1955. Wheat et al. reported the benefit of lowering blood pressure and aortic wall stress in the management and prevention of extension of aortic dissection in 1965.

Dissections of the aorta are clinically classified according to the part of aorta involved, regardless of the location of intimal tear. Two classifications that dictate the choice of therapy and prognosis of patients are the Stanford and the DeBakey classifications. Both systems are in use throughout the world. These classifications overlap somewhat; the Stanford A class includes the DeBakey classes I and II. Larson and Edward further classified DeBakey type III into IIIA, in which dissection originates beyond the left subclavian artery but extends both proximally and distally, and type IIIB, in which dissection extends distally.

The highest incidence of this disorder is reported in men 50–70 years of age. A history of hypertension is present in 70–90% of subjects. In persons younger than 40, dissection is usually associated with a familial predisposition to dissection; congenital disorders of connective tissue, such as Marfan syndrome and Ehlers-Danlos syndrome; and congenital lesions of the aorta. Half of dissections in women younger than 40 are associated with pregnancy. Nonpenetrating abdominal and chest trauma is another well-recognized, although unusual, cause of aortic dissection. Iatrogenic traumatic aortic dissections have occurred at the sites of aortic incisions, cross-clamping, cannulation, catheterization, and aortic valve replacement.

In 90% of cases, acute aortic dissection presents as sudden, severe chest pain in patients older than 50. The pain is typically described as excruciating, with a ripping, cutting, or tearing quality that is maximal at onset. Pain usually occurs in the anterior chest, may radiate to the interscapular area, and sometimes is present in the epigastric or lumbar regions, depending on the location and extent of dissection. Distal dissections more frequently present with back pain. With the propagation of medial hemorrhage, pain may migrate from its initial site to the neck, throat, jaw, or teeth, as occurs in ascending aortic dissections.

To prevent inappropriate institution of thrombolytic therapy, which can be hazardous to some patients (such as those with myocardial ischemia), pain due to dissection should be differentiated from chest pain resulting from other causes. The chest pain in acute myocardial infarction is said to be more gradual in onset and more heavy or crushing in character than the immediately intense tearing quality of aortic dissection. Examination for unequal pulses and asymmetric blood pressures provides important diagnostic clues for differentiating these two conditions. Aortic dissection is painless in approximately 12% of cases, particularly in patients with neurologic complications resulting from the dissection. Impairment of blood supply to the central nervous system may obtund a patients' perception of pain.

Hypotension is reported in up to 20% of cases with ascending aortic involvement. Blood pressure may be increased or decreased, and it may be different in each arm. Patients with aortic dissections may also present with dyspnea caused by associated congestive heart failure or with bronchospasm resulting from irritation of the left vagus nerve by a distorted aorta or rupture of a dissecting aorta into the pleural cavities or tracheobronchial tree. In some cases, a diastolic murmur of aortic regurgitation can be heard. Other new cardiac murmurs, systolic, diastolic, or both, may be present. Right atrial obstruction, rupture into the right atrium or right ventricle, and unexplained fever have been reported.

Compression of adjacent structures by the enlarged dissecting aorta or hemorrhage can cause various syndromes, such as Horner's syndrome (compression of the sympathetic chain), superior vena cava syndrome (caused by a distorted aorta, mediastinal hemorrhage, congestive heart failure, or cardiac tamponade), hoarseness (from recurrent laryngeal nerve compression), and dysphagia (caused by pressure on the esophagus from an enlarging aorta). A pulsatile sternoclavicular joint, although rarely present, may be a clue to the diagnosis. Acute aortic dissection may present similarly to ureteral colic, gastrointestinal disease, and peripheral vascular embolism. A pericardial friction rub, hemoptysis, hematemesis, and syncope are ominous signs that suggest aortic rupture.

Patients with suspected acute aortic dissection should be admitted to an ICU and placed under the care of an intensivist and a cardiovascular surgeon, if possible. Vascular pressures, urine output, mental status, and neurologic signs should be closely monitored for any deterioration caused by complications. IV antihypertensive treatment should be started in all patients (except patients with hypotension) as soon as the diagnosis of acute aortic dissection is suspected. The aim of antihypertensive therapy is to lessen the pulsatile load or aortic stress by lowering the blood pressure. Reducing the force of left ventricular contractions and, consequently, the rate at which the aortic pressure rises retards the propagation of the dissection and aortic rupture.

IV sodium nitroprusside is widely used to lower blood pressure in these cases because it is effective, easy to administer, and has a prompt onset of action. The infusion rate is adjusted so that a systolic blood pressure of 100–120 mm Hg is reached. Side effects such as nausea, hypotension, restlessness, and cyanide toxicity can occur if nitroprusside is used for extended periods, especially in patients with chronic renal insufficiency. Beta blockers are indicated for use with sodium nitroprusside, because sodium nitroprusside alone can cause an increase in the velocity of ventricular contraction and may lead to propagation of dissection. Bolus doses of IV propranolol are given, and a good response is indicated by a heart rate of 60–70 bpm. Esmolol, a short-acting beta-adrenergic antagonist, is alternative to propranolol. Labetalol, an alpha- and beta-adrenergic antagonist, is another alternative to the combination of nitroprusside and a beta blocker.

Cardiovascular surgical consultation is required in all patients with suspected aortic dissections. Surgery is indicated for all dissections involving the ascending aorta (Stanford type A dissection), except in those few patients with serious associated conditions that contraindicate surgery. Patients with hypotension that suggests aortic rupture are candidates for emergency surgical repair. Complications of Stanford type B dissections, such as leakage of blood from the aorta, impairment of blood flow to an organ or limb, or persistent pain despite an adequate medical regimen, are best treated by surgery. Younger patients with Marfan syndrome may benefit from surgery in the subacute phase and avoid rupture of a residual saccular aneurysm in the future.

The overall operative mortality rate for aortic dissections is 5–20%. Surgery in acute dissection is palliative rather than curative. The aim of surgery is to prevent rupture of the false lumen, re-establish blood flow in ischemic areas, and correct any associated acute aortic incompetence. The technique includes excising the part of the aorta with the intimal tear, obliterating entry into the false lumen proximally and distally, and inserting a prosthetic interposition graft. Incompetent valves can be reconstructed by resuspending the commissures, or, if that fails, a valve replacement may be considered. Surgical repair of the proximal aorta requires cardiopulmonary bypass, and deep hypothermia is used in arch repair in which circulatory arrest is necessary. Surgical outcome is based on factors such as age, severity of symptoms, postoperative organ dysfunction, and postoperative stroke.

Patients with uncomplicated distal dissections are best managed medically in the acute phase with antihypertensive therapy, because the survival rate is around 75% regardless of whether patients are treated medically or surgically. These patients are also generally older, with a history of cardiac, pulmonary, or renal diseases.

CLINICAL POINTS TO REMEMBER

1. Not all chest pain is ischemic in nature. Pulmonary embolism, aortic dissection, pneumothorax, and numerous other illnesses must be considered.

2. Predisposing conditions with abnormal tunica media (e.g., Marfan syndrome) should raise the clinician's index of suspicion for aortic dissection.

3. Despite the clinical course of our patient, thrombolysis is clearly not indicated in these cases.

SELECTED READINGS

Chen K, Varon J, Wenker O, et al. Acute aortic dissection: the basics. J Emerg Med 1997;15:859–867.

Edwards JE. Manifestations of acquired and congenital diseases of the aorta. Curr Probl Cardiol 1979;3:7–62.

Hirst AE, Gore I. The Etiology and Pathology of Aortic Dissection. In RM Doroghazi, EE Slater (eds), Aortic Dissection. New York: McGraw-Hill, 1983;13–53.

Marian AJ, Harris SL, Pickett JD, et al. Inadvertent administration of r-tPA to a patient with type I aortic dissection and subsequent cardiac tamponade. Am J Emerg Med 1993;11:613–615.

Roberts WC. Aortic dissection: anatomy, consequences and causes. Am Heart J 1981;101: 195–214.

13

An Elderly Lady with Urosepsis and an Intern's First Day in the Intensive Care Unit

On the evening of July 3, Mrs. M, an 86-year-old woman, is brought to the ICU with signs and symptoms consistent with a sepsis syndrome. After admission to the ICU, a thorough workup reveals that a urinary tract infection is the source of her sepsis. The patient becomes hemodynamically unstable and requires the placement of a pulmonary artery (Swan-Ganz) catheter.

Six hours later, the intern on call is summoned to Mrs. M's bedside because the patient's pulmonary artery tracing is "strange." On the basis of the tracing (Figure 13-1), the intern decides to advance the catheter. Mrs. M's mixed oxygen saturation, as demonstrated by the oximetric pulmonary artery catheter, is 90%. After two or three attempts to advance the catheter, the intern decides to leave it as it is and return to his bed to sleep. Five minutes later, the ICU fellow is called to see Mrs. M, who is now coughing up blood. When the fellow arrives at the bedside,

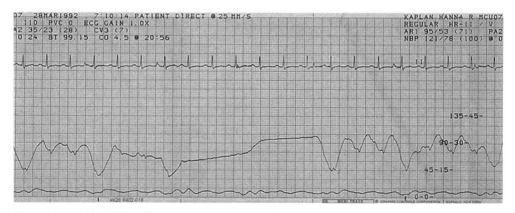

Figure 13-1 Mrs. M's pulmonary artery tracing when the intern was called to evaluate her.

Mrs. M is in severe respiratory distress and is emergently intubated. Active bleeding is noted coming from the endotracheal tube. Within 30 minutes, the patient dies, despite aggressive diagnostic and therapeutic maneuvers. Postmortem examination reveals a large tear in the right pulmonary artery.

DISCUSSION

This case is a classic presentation of a pulmonary artery catheter–induced pulmonary artery rupture. This uncommon complication of pulmonary artery catheterization occurs most frequently in patients that have oximetric pulmonary artery catheters, patients of advanced age, and patients with pulmonary artery abnormalities.

The case description makes it clear that the patient's pulmonary artery catheter was in the wedge position for some time before the intern's attempt to manipulate the catheter. He failed to recognize that the oxygen saturation was elevated and that the waveform was not compatible with a wedge tracing. At that point, the intern should have pulled back the pulmonary artery catheter instead of advancing it.

CLINICAL POINTS TO REMEMBER

1. Never advance a pulmonary artery catheter when unsure of its location.
2. An elevated oximetric reading in a patient with a pulmonary artery catheter may be the first indicator of a distal placement of the catheter and must be followed by pulling the catheter back promptly.
3. Patients with pulmonary artery catheters that remain in the wedge position for a significant period are prone to pulmonary artery ruptures.
4. The mortality rate for patients with pulmonary artery rupture is high.

SELECTED READINGS

Cokis C, Coombs L. Rupture of an abnormal pulmonary artery with a flow-directed pulmonary artery catheter. Anaesth Int Care 1997;25: 147–149.

Karak P, Dimick R, Hamrick KM, et al. Immediate transcatheter embolization of Swan-Ganz catheter-induced pulmonary artery pseudoaneurysm. Chest 1997;111:1450–1452.

Kearney TJ, Shabot MM. Pulmonary artery rupture associated with the Swan-Ganz catheter. Chest 1995;108:1349–1352.

Smart FW, Husserl FE. Complications of flow-directed balloon-tipped catheters. Chest 1990; 97:227–228.

14

A Nursing Student Gives Her First Sponge Bath

Mr. Jones is a 53-year-old businessman with a 60-pack-per-year smoking history. He presents with a 2-week history of intermittent hemoptysis and on evaluation is found to have a 5-cm squamous cell carcinoma involving the right pulmonary hilum. The metastatic workup is negative. Mediastinoscopy fails to reveal any nodal metastasis. Pulmonary function test demonstrates a forced expiratory volume in 1 second (FEV_1) of 78% of predicted, with a predicted postpneumonectomy FEV_1 of 1.2 liters.

Mr. Jones undergoes an exploratory right thoracotomy, during which the tumor is found to involve the truncus inferior of the right pulmonary artery and extend onto the pericardium in the region of the superior pulmonary vein. An intrapericardial pneumonectomy is performed to gain control of the superior pulmonary vein. The right pulmonary artery and inferior pulmonary vein are controlled outside the pericardium. The bronchial stump is covered with an intercostal muscle pedicle, and the defect in the pericardium is primarily closed with interrupted silk sutures. Air (900 cc) is aspirated from the right hemithorax, and the trachea is confirmed to be in a midline position by an intraoperative radiograph.

At the end of the operation, Mr. Jones is extubated and transferred to the ICU for postoperative monitoring. The estimated blood loss is only 150 ml. He remains in normal sinus rhythm with a heart rate between 70 and 90 bpm and systolic blood pressure of 120 mm Hg. His breath sounds are clear in the left lung, and a thoracic epidural catheter provides excellent pain control.

Mr. Jones is awake and alert while visiting with relatives during the regular ICU visiting hours that evening. He rests comfortably during the night, maintaining a urine output of 30 ml per hour and stable vital signs. During morning rounds, he is noted to have a low-grade temperature of 38.2°C and is slightly diaphoretic. The respiratory therapist continues to work with the patient sitting upright in bed and encourages him to use his incentive spirometer. He manages to expectorate a large mucus plug and feels much better.

The temperature persists, however, so a nursing student is asked to give the patient a sponge bath. The patient initially is rolled onto his left side. The dressing appears dry. The patient is then rolled onto his right side, and alcohol is applied. The monitor alarms! The nurse looks at the monitor and is shocked to see that the arterial pressure wave is dampened and shows a systolic pressure of only 30 mm Hg with severe bradycardia of 20 bpm. The patient is immediately repositioned on his back. He is now unconscious; taking deep, labored breaths; and showing intense venous congestion in his face and no improvement in his heart rate or blood pressure. The thoracic surgeon is paged at once and the ICU resident attempts to stabilize the patient with inotropics. A chest radiograph is taken.

The thoracic surgeon, who was about to start another case, arrives just as the radiology technician finishes taking the x-ray. The nurse quickly explains the patient's rapid deterioration after being placed in the right lateral decubitus position. The surgeon immediately asks for the emergency thoracotomy tray kept in the unit, positions the patient with his left side down, and emergently reopens the right hemithorax. The surgeon places his hand in the patient's chest, and within 10 seconds the patient regains his blood pressure.

DISCUSSION

Cardiac herniation is an immediate and life-threatening situation. It most commonly occurs after right pneumonectomies in which the pericardial sac is opened or a portion of it is resected. In this case, although the small defect was primarily repaired, a small cut in the pericardium was sufficient for the beating heart to linearly tear the defect and rotate on the superior vena cava–inferior vena cava (SVC-ICV) axis counterclockwise into the postpneumonectomy space on the right. The SVC-IVC axis is fixed, but the bulky and heavier left ventricle can be mobile and fall into the space. Rotation on the venous return axis results in immediate hypotension because the venous return is essentially cut off.

In such a case, all resuscitation efforts with fluids, inotropics, and open-chest cardiopulmonary resuscitation will fail, because the hypotension is related to mechanical occlusion of venous return. Occasionally, immediately moving the patient into a supine or left lateral decubitus position allows the heart to fall back into its normal anatomic position. If this does not occur, however, immediate reopening of the chest is required, with manual reduction of the heart into the pericardial sac. This usually must be done at the bedside based on clinical suspicion without even a confirming radiograph.

Any opening or resection of the right side of the pericardium during a pneumonectomy must be repaired with a synthetic mesh, usually made of Gore-Tex, Vicryl, or Marlex. If the entire posterior edge of the pericardium is resected, then the mesh must be reattached to the interatrial groove. The heart can shift into the left hemithorax without impeding venous return, so reconstruction on the left is not required. If a small opening is made, the best course may be to split the pericardium along its entire length or sew in a mesh (without tension), because a small defect can result in left ventricular herniation and in hypotension caused by a tourniquet effect on the left atrium. Cardiac herniation is not a problem if a portion of the lung remains on either side: An inflated lung buttresses the heart and prevents rotation into the postlobectomy space.

CLINICAL POINTS TO REMEMBER

1. Cardiac herniation is an immediate and life-threatening situation.
2. All resuscitation efforts with fluids, inotropics, and open-chest cardiopulmonary resuscitation will fail, because the hypotension is related to mechanical occlusion of venous return.
3. Occasionally, immediately moving the patient into a supine or left lateral decubitus position allows the heart to fall back into its normal anatomic position. If this does not occur, however, immediate reopening of the chest is required, with manual reduction of the heart into the pericardial sac. This usually must be done at the bedside based on clinical suspicion without even a confirming radiograph.

SELECTED READINGS

Bhalla M. Noncardiac thoracic surgical procedures. Definitions, indications, and postoperative radiology. Radiol Clin North Am 1996;34: 137–155.

Forget AP, Fleyfel M, Vallet B, et al. Cardiac herniation and subherniation. Complication of intrapericardial pneumonectomy. Ann Fr Anesth Reanim 1992;11:111–114.

Kirsh MM, Rotman H, Behrendt DM, et al. Complications of pulmonary resection. Ann Thorac Surg 1975;20:215–236.

15

A Young Head and Neck Resident and Her Clean White Coat

Rose has just completed her rotating surgical internship and is starting her first day as a head and neck surgical resident. She just picked up her new coat with her name proudly embossed over the pocket. Her pager goes off. A nurse on the postoperative head and neck surgical floor asks that she evaluate Mrs. Jones, a 46-year-old woman who had undergone a resection of benign vocal cord papillomas 5 days previously and has a prophylactic temporary tracheostomy in place to protect her airway from anticipated upper airway edema. Mrs. Jones is noted to have some fresh bleeding around the size-6 tracheostomy tube that had not been present previously.

On her arrival at the floor, the resident notes Mrs. Jones to be hemodynamically stable, with a heart rate of 72 bpm, and breathing comfortably at a rate of 14 breaths per minute. Mrs. Jones had a few coughing spells earlier this morning and noted about a tablespoon-full of bright red blood after one of these paroxysms. The bleeding appears to have slowed. The resident suspects that a small skin bleeder vessel or some granulation tissue is responsible for the bleeding.

Rose obtains a headlight from the operating room and some silver nitrate sticks. She cuts the ties that secure the tracheostomy and the anchoring skin sutures to permit examination around the tube. As the tube is rotated cephalad, an immediate massive hemorrhage occurs, bright red and under arterial pressure to the point that within 2 seconds Rose's coat is entirely covered in blood and blood has hit the wall behind her. The patient remains conscious but is now coughing violently.

DISCUSSION

A tracheoinnominate artery fistula is often a dramatic event that can result in the death of the patient. The major hemorrhage can be preceded by a small herald bleed that may be intermittent. The cause of such a fistula is related to the course of the innominate artery as it divides into the right subclavian and right common carotid arteries at an oblique angle close to the anterior wall of the trachea. In some patients, the innominate artery can ride up to or even occasionally above the level of the suprasternal notch. In other patients, a tracheostomy tube that is placed too low can result in mechanical contact between the rigid plastic tracheostomy tube and the soft superior margin of the innominate artery.

A combination of cephalocaudal movement of the trachea and larynx with respiratory motion and the arterial pulsation of the innominate artery can, even in a few days, result in a weakening and subsequent defect in the arterial wall with secondary tracheoinnominate artery fistulas. Local infection associated with all tracheostomies can also contribute to this. If a fistula is suspected and the clinical situation permits, an angiogram or careful bronchoscopic examination in the operating room with slow withdrawal of the tube in a controlled environment can be performed.

An unsuspecting surgical resident faced with an emergency situation like the one described here must have a well thought-out plan to deal with this condition. Two aspects of this emergency take priority: (1) maintenance of the airway and (2) control of the massive hemorrhage. One possible maneuver involves forcibly retracting the tracheostomy tube anteriorly with overinflation of the cuff of the tracheostomy to compress the innominate artery between the tube and the posterior aspect of the manubrium. If this is not possible, replacement of the tracheostomy tube with an endotracheal tube passed distally and digitally to compress the innominate artery against the posterior table of the manubrium can temporarily control the hemorrhage. Provisions must be made for transporting the patient immediately to the operating room, and blood products must be rapidly obtained. In the operating room, a thoracic surgeon should divide the sternum and, in most cases, ligate the innominate artery, attempt repair of the tracheal stoma, and interpose autologous tissue in the area of the repair.

Primary repair of the artery or grafting must be discouraged in this contaminated field, because it will certainly result in future dehiscence of the repair. Although a cerebral vascular accident may result from proximal innominate artery ligation, most patients have sufficient collateralization to prevent this. An understanding of the etiology and anatomy involved permits a quick response to this rare but often lethal complication.

CLINICAL POINTS TO REMEMBER

1. Tracheoinnominate artery fistulas are often dramatic events that can result in the death of the patient.
2. If a fistula is suspected and the clinical situation permits, an angiogram or careful bronchoscopic examination in the operating room with slow withdrawal of the tube in a controlled environment can be performed.
3. Provisions must be made for transporting the patient immediately to the operating room.
4. Maintenance of a patent airway is paramount in the management of these patients.

SELECTED READINGS

Alfaro J, Varela G, DeMiguel E, Martin de Nicolas JL. Successful management of a tracheoinnominate artery fistula following placement of a wire self-expandable tracheal Gianturco stent. Eur J Cardiothorac Surg 1993;7:615–616.

Gelman JJ, Aro M, Weiss SM. Tracheoinnominate artery fistula. J Am Coll Surg 1994;179:626–634.

Nelems JM. Tracheoinnominate artery fistula. Am J Surg 1981;141:526–527.

16

Crazy as a Loon and Peeing Like a Race Horse

The sun is beating down brightly on the Gulf Coast region of Texas. An ED receives a telephone call indicating that a helicopter is on its way from an offshore oil platform. Apparently, an offshore worker fell into the void tank and had to be rescued by coworkers. The patient was observed to have aspirated large quantities of the fluid in the tank.

After his rescue, the patient's mental status began to deteriorate and he started urinating excessively. He is transported by helicopter to the ED. On arrival, the patient is confused, chest and abdominal examinations demonstrate that he is tachycardic to a rate of 135 bpm, and his respiratory rate is 18 breaths per minute. The only other pertinent information gathered from physical examination is evidence of minimal trauma to the head, with a small laceration or abrasion of the frontal region. The patient produces approximately 1 liter of urine during the first 30 minutes of his ED stay.

Given the changes in mental status, a routine metabolic profile is investigated and a CT scan of the head performed. Both investigations are within normal limits. Serum calcium level measured at 20 mg/dl. The patient is treated with saline diuresis, and a rapid reduction in his calcium level and improvement in his mental status and polyuria are achieved.

DISCUSSION

Changes in mental status suggest a number of different clinical conditions. Structural lesions of the central nervous system must be considered in any victim of trauma. However, a broad range of metabolic abnormalities may result in mental status changes.

The victim described in this case report had fallen into a tank on a offshore drilling platform. Calcium salts are used for many purposes in the drilling and completion process, and high concentrations of calcium may be present in certain drilling fluids. This patient was presumed to have aspirated a small but significant quantity of solutions with a high calcium content, which led to his hypercalcemia and the subsequent mental status changes and polyuria.

Other kinds of environments and near-drowning may produce a similar phenomenon. It has been described in near-drownings in the Dead Sea and several other lakes with high calcium contents scattered around the globe.

CLINICAL POINTS TO REMEMBER

1. Consider metabolic derangement in all patients who present with altered mental status.
2. Toxic exposures may occur in industrial settings, and even common industrial chemicals may produce intoxication.
3. In cases of near-drowning, the constituents of the drowning fluid must be determined, because profound electrolyte abnormalities have been observed in high solute concentration exposures.

SELECTED READING

Fromm RE. Hypercalcemia complicating an industrial near drowning. Ann Emerg Med 1991;20: 669–671.

17

The Snake Charmer with Shortness of Breath

Pedro, a 19-year-old man, works as a gardener in an affluent neighborhood in Houston, Texas. A diligent worker, he spends a lot of time cleaning flower beds on the grounds of the large homes in the neighborhood. While preparing a bed in the corner of a yard that abuts an open field, he encounters a small snake. Having spent his life in the outdoors, Pedro has encountered a number of reptiles and thus is unafraid of this new acquaintance. In fact, he is fascinated by this particular snake, which he nicknames "Chiquita." He picks it up for a closer examination. Juan, who is Pedro's coworker, sees the rattles at the end of the snake's tail and yells at Pedro to "drop the viper." Pedro tells him that this is only a "baby snake" and that he is "a man," and "can handle it." Shortly thereafter, the snake decides otherwise and bites Pedro on the dorsum of the right hand. Juan grabs his shovel and proceeds to "charm" the snake by repeatedly striking it with the blade of the garden implement.

Pedro is in pain, and Juan scoops up the snake and his friend, tumbles them into the pickup truck, and heads to the local ED. On arrival at the ED, Pedro complains of severe pain and swelling in his right hand and a bad case of "stupidity." He is mildly tachycardic (105 bpm) with blood pressure of 140/90 mm Hg and a respiratory rate of 18 breaths per minute. His physical examination is unremarkable, except for the site of envenomation (Figure 17-1). Two puncture wounds are seen in the middle of significant swelling and erythema that encompass the whole of the right hand and extend into the wrist.

The snake is examined by the ED physician, and its rattles are quickly identified (Figure 17-2). Out of concern over the local appearance of the wound, the ED physician administers antivenin. Within 10 minutes of administration of the antivenin, Pedro begins to complain of shortness of breath. A second physical examination reveals moderate respiratory distress manifested by tachypnea. Substantial facial swelling is also noted, with mild to moderate inspiratory stridor (Figure 17-3). Antihistamines and corticosteroids are administered, and Pedro is transferred to the ICU.

In the ICU, Pedro develops mild renal dysfunction with evidence of rhabdomyolysis and requires debridement of the wound. Within a few days, he has improved and is discharged home. Pedro asks for what is left of "Chiquita" and now has a new snakeskin belt.

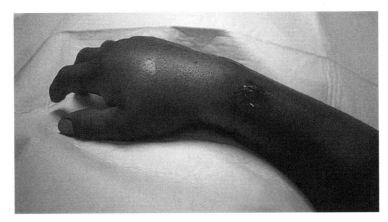

Figure 17-1   When Pedro arrived at the emergency department, his hand was swollen and two puncture wounds were evident.

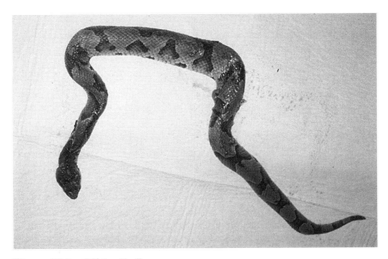

Figure 17-2   "Chiquita."

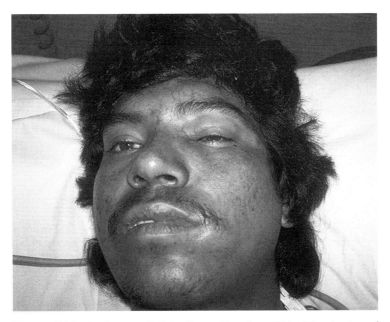

Figure 17-3 Pedro reacted to the antivenin within 10 minutes of administration.

DISCUSSION

Poisonous snakes reside in many regions of the United States, although most bites occur in the Southern and Southwestern states. Approximately 8,000 instances of poisonous snakebite occur annually in the United States; however, only 9–15 deaths result. The peak incidence is during the summer months. Four groups of venomous snake species are found in the United States: rattlesnakes (genus *Crotalus* and *Sistrurus*), copperheads (*Agkistrodon contortrix*), and cottonmouths (*Agkistrodon piscivorus*)—all of which are pit vipers—and coral snakes (genus *Micrurus*). Rattlesnakes account for 65% of reported venomous snake bites.

Snake venoms are complex mixtures of toxins that have cytotoxic, hemotoxic, and neurotoxic components. Cytotoxic effects produce tissue necrosis. Hemotoxic venoms interfere with the coagulation system. Rattlesnakes traditionally are thought to have cytotoxic and hemotoxic venom, but neurotoxic activity may also be present. Coral snake venom has largely neurotoxic activity. Snakes are capable of controlling the quantity of venom administered, and approximately 25–30% of poisonous snakebites do not result in envenomation.

The management of snakebite remains controversial. Equine antivenin is available for many pit vipers. Crotalid-polyvalent antivenin has been recommended by some authors for pit viper envenomations. Skin-testing for horse serum sensitivity is recommended before administration (it was not done in this case). The dosage of antivenin recommended is determined by the severity of the envenomation. Research on antivenins is scarce, but some efficacy for hemostatic abnormalities and shock is reported. Antivenins usually fail to prevent renal injury and local necrosis.

Although little agreement exists on treatment for snakebite, what should not be done is well established. Icing or cooling the bite is not recommended, because it may actually be harmful. Tourniquets should be avoided, and no incisions should be made over the wound; these measures have not proved useful and may cause further injury.

Pedro's case was complicated by a generalized anaphylactic reaction. The onset of anaphylaxis varies from individual to individual, as does the severity. Upper airway obstruction as a consequence of edema of the larynx and swelling of the tongue and lips may result in stridor and asphyxia. The management of patients with anaphylaxis consists of assessing and securing the airway, breathing, and circulation. Epinephrine is the drug of choice for these patients. Antihistamines and corticosteroids are also used.

CLINICAL POINTS TO REMEMBER

1. Most victims of snakebite are male and younger than 20 years.
2. The most important findings for pit viper envenomation are fang punctures at the bite site (usually on the extremities), local pain, and adjacent erythema and edema.
3. Anaphylactic reactions can occur after administration of an antivenin.
4. If antivenin is to be given, skin-testing for horse serum sensitivity should be done first.

SELECTED READINGS

Dart RC, Seifert SA, Carroll L, et al. Affinity-purified, mixed monospecific crotalid antivenom ovine Fab for the treatment of crotalid venom poisoning. Ann Emerg Med 1997;30:33–39.

Moss ST, Bogdan G, Dart RC, et al. Association of rattlesnake bite location with severity of clinical manifestations. Ann Emerg Med 1997;30:58–61.

Sternbach GL, Varon J. Environmental Disorders. In J Varon (ed), Practical Guide to the Care of the Critically Ill Patient. St. Louis: Mosby–Year Book, 1994;125–148.

18

The Revenge of the Barbecue Grill

Peter, John, Robert, and JoAnn (members of the same household) present to the ED, all complaining of headache, lethargy, abdominal cramping, and nausea. They relate a history of drinking unrefrigerated milk on the evening before presentation. Peter and John have mild orthostatic blood pressure changes. They are treated with IV fluids and discharged with a diagnosis of infectious gastroenteritis. Robert remains in the ED with persistent symptoms. Several hours later, four other members of the same family present to the ED with similar complaints. They are evaluated and treated with IV fluids, and all are discharged, including Robert.

Several hours later, Leticia, Mary, Joseph, and Ramon (more members of the same family) present to the ED with similar complaints. Mary had not ingested the suspected milk, but she suffers from migraine headache and feels that her symptoms are associated with one of her headaches. Specific questions about home heating systems do not suggest mechanical problems; in fact, the heating system was not in use. An unaffected relative who lives elsewhere admits to cooking indoors with charcoal briquettes in the barbecue grill, after originally claiming that the cooking was done outdoors.

Arterial blood samples are drawn and sent for carboxyhemoglobin (COHb) testing. The results in each patient are 6.9%, 15.1%, 27.1%, and 37.4%. The two patients with lower COHb levels are treated with 100% oxygen in the ED for 2 hours and show symptomatic improvement. The other two patients are admitted to the ICU. The fire department is deployed to check the house and reports a barbecue grill in the middle of the living room and evidence of smoke damage.

DISCUSSION

This case illustrates the importance of always considering carbon monoxide (CO) poisoning when two or more patients are similarly or simultaneously sick. The diagnosis must be excluded by the taking of a directed history and by physical examination.

CO is the leading cause of death by poisoning in the United States. It is also the most common cause of death in combustion-related inhalation injury. CO combines preferentially with hemoglobin to produce COHb, displacing oxygen and reducing systemic arterial oxygen (O_2) content. Dissolved CO delivered to tissues, especially to the heart and brain, causes most of the CO toxicity by binding with the cytochrome a_3. Dissolved CO, therefore, not COHb, causes toxicity.

In room air, the half-life of COHb is 320 minutes in young, healthy volunteers. Administration of 100% O_2 at 1 atm reduces the half-life to 80.3 minutes, and 100% O_2 at 3 atm reduces the half-life to 23.3 minutes. CO binds to cardiac and skeletal myoglobin as well as to hemoglobin. Cardiac myoglobin binds three times more CO than skeletal myoglobin. Because of carboxymyoglobin's higher affinity for myoglobin, carboxymyoglobin is slower to dissociate than COHb, and a rebound effect with delayed return of symptoms may be seen.

CO poisoning does not cause dyspnea or tachypnea until hypoxemia from circulatory dysfunction or lactic acidosis from tissue hypoxia sets in. At low levels, chronic cardiopulmonary problems (e.g., angina and chronic obstructive pulmonary disease) may be exacerbated because cardiac myoglobin binds with great affinity and rapidly reduces myocardial O_2 reserves.

With acute exposure, blood levels correlate with symptoms and signs but do not reflect tissue CO levels. Arterial blood gases are used to determine the degree of CO intoxication and the level of treatment necessary. With COHb levels lower than 10%, the patient is usually asymptomatic. As COHb rises above 20%, the patient may develop headache, dizziness, confusion, and nausea. Chest pain caused by myocardial ischemia may occur, as may cardiac arrhythmias. Coma and seizures resulting from cerebral edema are common with levels higher than 40%, and death is likely at levels higher than 60%.

The mainstays of therapy are supplemental O_2 and monitoring for cardiac dysrhythmias. The goal of O_2 therapy is to improve the O_2 content of the blood by maximizing the fraction dissolved in plasma. The advantage of administering hyperbaric O_2 is a more rapid reduction in COHb levels. Disadvantages of this treatment include the scarcity of available treatment centers and the necessity of patient transport. Patients with severe neurologic or cardiovascular symptoms or very high COHb levels will benefit from hyperbaric O_2; however, transportation is most hazardous for these very sick patients. Once treatment begins, O_2 therapy and observation must continue long enough to rule out delayed sequelae as the carboxymyoglobin unloads.

The differential diagnosis for CO poisoning includes viral illnesses, food poisoning, depression, transient ischemic attacks, coronary artery disease, arrhythmias, and functional illnesses, among others. The most common misdiagnosis is a flu-like syndrome. The initial presentation of the patients in this case was consistent with gastroenteritis, for which they were given IV hydration and other supportive measures. Inhaled toxins initially were not considered. Once an adequate history, which included indoor cooking, and arterial blood gas results were obtained, the patients were placed on 100% O_2 with complete resolution of their symptoms.

CLINICAL POINTS TO REMEMBER

1. Consider CO poisoning when two or more patients are similarly or simultaneously sick.
2. The diagnosis of CO poisoning must be excluded by a directed history and physical examination.
3. With acute exposure, blood levels correlate with symptoms and signs but do not reflect tissue CO levels.
4. The differential diagnosis of CO poisoning includes viral illnesses, food poisoning, depression, transient ischemic attacks, coronary artery disease, dysrhythmias,

and functional illnesses, among others. The most common misdiagnosis is a flu-like syndrome.

SELECTED READINGS

Anderson GK. Treatment of carbon monoxide poisoning with hyperbaric oxygen. Mil Med 1978;143:538–541.

Gasman JD, Varon J, Gardner J. The revenge of the barbecue grill: carbon monoxide poisoning. West J Med 1990;153:656–657.

Heimbach DM, Waeckerle JF. Inhalation injuries. Ann Emerg Med 1988;17:1316–1320.

Meredith T, Vale A. Carbon monoxide poisoning. BMJ 1988;296:77–79.

Myers RA, Linberg SE, Cowley RA. Carbon monoxide poisoning: the injury and its treatment. JACEP 1979;8:479–484.

Sadovnikoff N, Varon J, Sternbach GL. Carbon monoxide poisoning: an occult epidemic. Postgrad Med 1992;92:86–96.

19

Hemodynamic Collapse in a Smoker and the New Respiratory Therapist

Roscoe is a 62-year-old man with a passion for cigarettes and football. He has been feeling unwell for the last 4 or 5 days, but, given that it is football season, he has not taken the time to see his physician. When he finally presents to his doctor's office, he is acutely ill, with a cough productive of yellow sputum, fever to 38.5°C, and chills. He is admitted directly to the medicine floor. Initial treatment consists of the administration of inhaled bronchodilators by hand-held nebulizer, IV antibiotics, and supplemental O_2. Roscoe deteriorates rapidly; he becomes lethargic and requires intubation and assisted mechanical ventilation.

Jim-Bob, a new hire in the respiratory therapy department, is delegated to set up the mechanical ventilator. As he approaches the ventilator, he recognizes his football buddy Roscoe and asks him, "What happened to you, man?" Roscoe indicates with his hand that he is not getting enough air, and Jim-Bob, in accordance with the standing orders of the institution, increases the respiratory rate within the specified range.

Ten minutes later, the ICU nurse summons the physician on call to Roscoe's bedside. Roscoe's blood pressure has fallen from 140/76 to 70/40 mm Hg. The physician begins an infusion of dopamine. Roscoe's blood pressure continues to fall, despite high doses of dopamine. Simultaneously, Jim-Bob, who is present at the bedside, notes that the airway pressures have risen and recommends a chest radiograph to rule out a pneumothorax. The physician on call is concerned that secretions may be occluding the endotracheal tube and asks that the patient be suctioned. On disconnection from the mechanical ventilator and suctioning, Roscoe's blood pressure begins to rise and a small amount of thick secretion is obtained. The physician on call, proud of his diagnostic acumen, has Roscoe reconnected to the mechanical ventilator. Jim-Bob observes a repeat decline in Roscoe's blood pressure shortly after the institution of mechanical ventilation. Roscoe has a cardiopulmonary arrest within minutes, and the code team arrives. He is disconnected from mechanical ventilation to be manually ventilated and responds promptly to resuscitative efforts. A quick review of the ventilator settings and events that occurred leads the critical care fellow to the correct diagnosis.

DISCUSSION

Hemodynamic compromise after the institution of mechanical ventilation suggests a number of diagnostic possibilities. The underlying pathology that leads to the need for mechanical ventilation may be responsible for hypotension. However, the clinician must be constantly aware of the possibility that complications of mechanical ventilation itself may produce cardiovascular collapse. Major considerations include pneumothorax, hypoxemia, hypercarbia, and intrinsic positive end-expiratory pressure (auto-PEEP).

Auto-PEEP is the phenomena whereby functional residual capacity increases because of incomplete exhalation, as when there is inadequate time for complete exhalation to occur. Extrinsic PEEP is the pressure applied to the airways by the clinician. Total PEEP is the pressure measured when all flow is stopped at the end of expiration. Thus,

total PEEP = extrinsic PEEP + auto-PEEP.

Several factors produce auto-PEEP: Increased airway resistance predisposes to the development of auto-PEEP, as does a decrease in expiratory time, usually produced by an increase in respiratory rate.

Manifestations of auto-PEEP include declining blood pressure, due to impairment of venous return, and rising airway pressures. Simply examining expiratory pressure on the mechanical ventilator pressure monitoring device does not reveal the presence of auto-PEEP. Occlusion of the expiratory circuit at the end of expiration is one way of measuring the level of auto-PEEP. Examining flow waveforms may also suggest auto-PEEP, because expiratory flow does not approach zero before inspiration begins. Roscoe's clinical picture is a classic example of a patient with pre-existing obstructive lung disease and dynamic hyperinflation that are exacerbated by a shortened expiratory time. The inexperienced respiratory care practitioner, hoping to relieve the discomfort of his friend and patient, actually contributed to his near-death. Roscoe was literally blown up like a football.

The management of patients with auto-PEEP is simple and requires prolongation of expiratory time. Removing the patient from the mechanical ventilator results, in most instances, in prompt improvement of the hemodynamic status. Reinstitution of mechanical ventilation with increased expiratory time (usually accomplished by decreasing respiratory rate) corrects the problem. Unrecognized auto-PEEP may lead to profound cardiovascular collapse and even cardiac arrest.

CLINICAL POINTS TO REMEMBER

1. Patients on mechanical ventilation who develop hemodynamic compromise should be evaluated for complications of the mechanical ventilation.
2. Assessment for the presence of auto-PEEP (i.e., measurement of end-expiratory static pressures) should be part of the initial assessment.
3. Prolonging expiratory time is the therapeutic response to excessive auto-PEEP.
4. Volume expansion and other methods of improving venous return may also help.

SELECTED READINGS

Keith RL, Pierson DJ. Complications of mechanical ventilation. A bedside approach. Clin Chest Med 1996;17:439–451.

Ranieri VM, Grasso S, Fiore T, Giuliani R. Autopositive end-expiratory pressure and dynamic hyperinflation. Clin Chest Med 1996;17:379–394.

Ranieri VM, Dambrosio M, Brienza N. Intrinsic PEEP and cardiopulmonary interaction in patients with COPD and acute ventilatory failure. Eur Respir J 1996;9:1283–1292.

Rossi A, Polese G, Brandi G, Conti G. Intrinsic positive end-expiratory pressure (PEEPi). Intensive Care Med 1995;21:522–536.

20

New Murmur and Collapse in an Investment Banker Admitted to the Coronary Care Unit

Andrew is a 38-year-old investment banker who has been under a fair amount of stress recently because of changes in Pacific Rim stocks. He has been spending a number of late nights in meetings and drinking a fair amount of coffee. In the middle of the night, his wife becomes concerned that he does not look well and calls emergency medical services (911). Andrew is brought to a local ED, where an ECG demonstrates changes consistent with an anterolateral infarction. He is treated with thrombolysis, and improvement in the ECG changes is noted. He is admitted for observation to the coronary care unit.

The next morning, he is noted to have shortness of breath, and on examination a loud systolic murmur is heard along the left sternal border. A pulmonary artery (Swan-Ganz) catheter is placed, which demonstrates a step-up in the O_2 saturation from the right atrium to the pulmonary artery. A presumed diagnosis of an acute ventricular septal defect is made. Andrew continues to deteriorate and requires replacement of the intra-aortic balloon pump. After he is stabilized, he is transferred to the cardiac surgical suite.

DISCUSSION

Myocardial infarction (MI) remains the major cause of morbidity and mortality in the United States, with approximately 1.2 million acute MIs and more than 400,000 resulting deaths each year. Mortality occurs in a number of different ways, but typically dysrhythmias and pump dysfunction (congestive heart failure) are at fault.

Mechanical complications of acute MI are not frequent but vigilance is required of the intensivist if appropriate management is to follow. These mechanical complications include ventricular septal rupture, manifested by the development of a new murmur and rapid progression of congestive heart failure; papillary muscle rupture, also manifested by the development of progressive heart failure associated with murmur onset; and free wall rupture, which may progress to cardiac tamponade and death.

Improvements in our understanding of the appropriate management of these patients have led to rapid repair of patients with ventricular septal rupture in response to attempts to improve morbidity and mortality before the complications of a prolonged period of congestive heart failure ensue.

CLINICAL POINTS TO REMEMBER

1. The development of a new murmur in patients with MI must prompt aggressive efforts at diagnosis and therapy if optimal management is to be ensured.
2. Early surgical intervention in the mechanical complications of MI should be considered.
3. Noninvasive diagnostic techniques, in particular Doppler echocardiography and color-flow Doppler imaging, have greatly improved our ability to make the diagnosis of mechanical complications in the early phases of MI.

SELECTED READINGS

Montoya A, McKeever L, Scanlon P, et al. Early repair of ventricular septal rupture after infarction. Am J Cardiol 1980;45:345–348.

Skillington PD, Davies RH, Luff AJ, et al. Surgical treatment for infarct-related ventricular septal defects: improved early results combined with analysis of late functional status. J Thorac Cardiovasc Surg 1990;99:798–808.

21

The Canadian Corpse Who Wiggled Her Toes

It is a snowy Valentine's Day in Toronto, Ontario. Sarah tries to contact her 64-year-old mother, who lives next door, by phone, but the mother does not answer. Sarah puts on her ski jacket, runs next door in the –20°C weather, and lets herself into her mother's house. She notices that it is cold and finds her mother sitting in a recliner in the living room, with a glass of wine on the side table in front of the fireplace. The embers are low, and it appears that her mother has fallen asleep in the chair. Sarah tries to wake her, but she is cold, stiff, and unresponsive. She appears to be dead.

Emergency medical services and the family physician are called immediately. When they arrive, the physician pronounces the patient dead and the body is transported to a local hospital morgue. The mother is suspected of having suffered a fatal cardiovascular event.

While the corpse is in the hallway of the morgue, a passing janitor notes that one of her toes appears to move slowly. Terrified, he notifies the pathology technician, who corroborates the finding. Together, they rush the corpse upstairs to the ED. On arrival at the ED, a senior nurse detects a palpable but barely discernible central pulse of 8 bpm. After the patient is transferred to the emergency stretcher, the pulse disappears. No recordable blood pressure or spontaneous respiration is observed. The patient's core body temperature is measured at 26°C via a rectal probe. CPR is initiated, including intubation and assisted ventilation. An immediate cardiothoracic surgical consultation is requested for active core rewarming with cardiopulmonary bypass. A monitor strip obtained at that time is depicted in Figure 21-1.

An attempt at electrical defibrillation is made without success. While CPR is continued, active core rewarming is started via percutaneous femorofemoral extracorporeal bypass. After 20 minutes of active core rewarming, the patient spontaneously converts to a sinus bradycardia with a central carotid pulse of 40 bpm, and CPR is stopped. For the next 30 minutes, active core rewarming is continued. The patient's core temperature rises to 35°C. At this time, a palpable peripheral pulse is felt, with a recordable blood pressure of 80/40 mm Hg and a heart rate of 52 bpm. Once the patient becomes normothermic and normotensive, she is weaned from the extracorporeal circuit and transported the ICU, where she continues to make an uneventful recovery without neurologic complications.

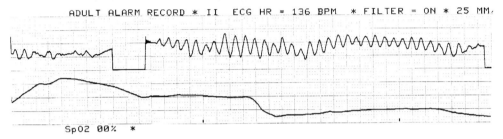

Figure 21-1   The patient's monitor strip immediately after the loss of a palpable pulse.

DISCUSSION

This case underscores the danger of overlooking a diagnosis of profound hypothermia in an elderly patient. Hypothermia is commonly defined as a core body temperature below 35°C. A more detailed scheme divides hypothermia into four levels: mild hypothermia, with a core temperature between 34.0° and 36.5°C; moderate hypothermia, with a core temperature from 28° to 34°C; deep hypothermia, with a core temperature between 17° and 28°C; and profound hypothermia, with a core temperature from 4° to 17°C. The incidence of hypothermia is probably underestimated; standard clinical thermometers do not measure low temperatures, and no uniform reporting systems exist. These factors lead to one of the most common errors in the management of hypothermia, the failure to recognize its presence. The majority of victims of cold have a subtle presentation, with the diagnosis being made incidentally after a routine temperature is obtained. Clinical manifestation may be as mild as confusion, in an elderly patient, or as dramatic as unconsciousness or even the simulation of death.

Primary (or accidental) hypothermia is caused by sufficiently prolonged exposure to a low environmental temperature that normal heat conservation mechanisms cannot overcome. However, extreme cold is by no means a prerequisite to the development of accidental hypothermia. Patients exposed to a modestly cold environment (10–15°C) for prolonged periods may develop severe hypothermia. Secondary hypothermia arises when heat conservation mechanisms are abnormal as a consequence of underlying disease. In secondary hypothermia, there may be an interference between the hypothalamic temperature-regulating center or the patient's capacity to shiver, redistribute blood, or move out of the cold environment.

Initial management of hypothermia should include general resuscitative measures and concomitant rewarming. General measures entail standard basic life support protocols, including obtaining adequate airway, breathing, and circulation (the ABCs). CPR should be initiated when indicated and should not be discontinued until a core temperature of 32°C has been reached without cardiac response. Patients in ventricular fibrillation are unlikely to respond to electrical defibrillation if their core temperature is below 30°C. Lidocaine may be effective, but bretylium has been recommended as the drug of choice for hypothermia-related ventricular fibrillation. A single attempt may be made at defibrillation, but if this is unsuccessful, efforts should be directed at circulatory support until the core temperature is higher than 30°C before defibrillation is tried again.

Rewarming techniques can be divided in three general modalities: passive rewarming, active surface rewarming, and active core rewarming. Passive rewarming involves removing the patient from the cold environment and applying dry, unheated blankets. This approach should be used in all hypothermic patients, at least initially. Passive rewarming is frequently sufficient in mild hypothermia when more rapid rewarming techniques are not indicated. Most cases of secondary hypothermia fall into this category, and passive rewarming should be accompanied by treatment of the underlying medical disorder.

Active surface rewarming involves the application of external sources of warmth to the body surfaces, such as heating blankets, hot water bottles, warm water (by immersion), heat cradles or, in one report, a heated, fluidized bead bed. With the exception of the last, these methods are usually readily available and noninvasive, but they are associated with a number of potential complications. An initial afterdrop in core temperature may be seen as peripheral vasoconstriction reverses and blood circulates through cold extremities. Although trunk-only warming techniques have been used to prevent this phenomenon, no advantage has been demonstrated over whole-body rewarming. In addition, rapid vasodilation may precipitate hypovolemic shock if the patient has undergone cold diuresis and fluid resuscitation has been inadequate. Immersion techniques are cumbersome and may impair monitoring and resuscitative efforts.

Active core rewarming has become the method of choice for all but mild hypothermia and is absolutely indicated for patients in ventricular fibrillation. Core rewarming techniques are invasive and involve significantly greater risks, but the rate of rewarming is substantially faster, and survival rates for most techniques are better than with surface methods. Core rewarming techniques include infusion of warmed IV fluids, inhalation of warmed respiratory gases, hemodialysis, peritoneal dialysis, enteral irrigation, and extracorporeal blood rewarming.

Warmed IV fluids are easily administered and treat both the hypothermia and associated hypovolemia, but their temperature must not exceed 40°C, and the induced rate of core temperature rise is therefore modest. Warmed, humidified gas administration takes advantage of the large surface area of the alveoli for use as a heat exchanger, and it is a relatively benign intervention, as long as the airway temperature is maintained at less than 45°C to avoid thermal airway injury. Hemodialysis is very effective and especially valuable in patients with concomitant drug ingestion, but it requires specialized personnel and equipment and carries a risk of aggravating hypotension as well as the usual risks of hemodialysis. Peritoneal dialysis is practical and effective, with normothermia usually accomplished by six to eight exchanges of potassium-free dialysate heated to 43°C.

Gastric irrigation with placement of an intragastric balloon is a practical means of instilling warmed fluids but may provoke dysrhythmias. High colonic irrigation may be used, but it is less practical than peritoneal lavage, because smaller volumes of liquid are used and fecal obstruction or failure of retention may defeat the procedure. Mediastinal irrigation is highly invasive and must be performed in the operating room; it is, therefore, rarely used.

Extracorporeal blood rewarming may be performed by heating blood shunted from the femoral artery to the femoral vein to 40°C with a heat exchanger, as described in this case. This is relatively easily accomplished, may be performed without heparin, and is felt by many to be the treatment of choice for severe hypothermia.

Dysrhythmias are least frequently seen in ethanol-intoxicated hypothermic patients, which has led some individuals to propose that ethanol has a cardioprotective effect. The presence of vital signs on first contact is a favorable indicator. Markedly elevated potassium and ammonia levels denote cell lysis and are predictors of a fatal outcome.

CLINICAL POINTS TO REMEMBER

1. Although hypothermia is a serious and sometimes fatal condition, the prompt recognition of this entity and the institution of appropriate rewarming techniques may revive even profoundly affected individuals.
2. Many patients have been successfully resuscitated from profound levels of hypothermia. This has given rise to the dictum, "No patient is dead until warm and dead." The physician should not be guided by this away from the recognition that hypothermia is a frequently overlooked and potentially devastating syndrome in which prompt institution of therapy is needed to prevent serious consequences.

SELECTED READINGS

Danzl D. Accidental Hypothermia. In P Rosen (ed), Emergency Medicine. St. Louis: Mosby, 1988; 663–692.

Danzl D, Pozos R, Auerbach P, et al. Multicenter hypothermia survey. Ann Emerg Med 1987;16: 104–255.

Tolman K, Cohen A. Accidental hypothermia. Can Med Assoc J 1970;103:1357–1360.

Varon J, Sadovnikoff N, Sternbach GL. Hypothermia: saving patients from the big chill. Postgrad Med 1992;92:47–59.

22

Who Turned the Mediastinoscope Light Off?

Mrs. Jones is a 65-year-old woman who has been referred to Elsewhere General for the evaluation of a large right upper lobe tumor suspicious for bronchogenic cancer. A CT scan shows that she has several enlarged mediastinal nodes (N2 and N3) suspicious for metastatic disease. She is referred to young Dr. L, who has recently started his thoracic surgery practice.

Mrs. Jones is scheduled to have her elective staging mediastinoscopy late one Wednesday afternoon. She is anesthetized, and a fiberoptic bronchoscopy is performed, with normal findings. She is positioned for mediastinoscopy with a roll between her shoulders and her neck extended. A 3-cm incision is made a finger's breadth above her sternal notch and deepened through the platysma muscle; the strap muscles are divided in the midline. The pretracheal fascia is incised, and initial blunt digital dissection is performed immediately above the trachea, opening a space beneath her innominate artery. Firm but mobile right- and left-sided paratracheal nodes are palpated. The mediastinoscope is inserted. A large right paratracheal node (station 4R) just proximal to the right mainstem bronchus is identified. The node appears free in the lumen of the mediastinoscope. A large biopsy forceps is used to biopsy this node. On biopsy of the node, visualization through the mediastinoscope is lost, and Dr. L immediately turns his head to see if the fiberoptic light cord has been disconnected. When he turns back to examine the patient, a large amount of dark blue blood is pouring out of the mediastinoscope. The mediastinum is packed with gauze for 10 minutes, and the patient is typed and crossed for 6 units of blood. After 10 minutes the packing is removed. Again, a large amount of dark blood drains from the wound. The mediastinum is tightly packed once more and preparations are made for an emergency thoracotomy to repair an injury to a major vascular structure.

DISCUSSION

The three-dimensional anatomy of the thorax and mediastinum is quite complex. Although serious complications are reported in the literature in less than 0.5% of performances of this staging procedure, at one time or another all major vascular structures in the superior mediastinum have been injured during elective mediastinoscopy. Vessels at greatest risk include the innominate artery, the bottom of the ascending aorta, the top of the right main pulmonary artery (truncus anterior), the azygos vein, and small bronchial and subcarinal arteries that can also bleed profusely. Lymph nodes should be needle-aspirated before biopsy to ensure that what is perceived as nodal tissue is in fact not a vascular structure or that the lymph node itself is not densely adherent to an underlying vessel. Constant anatomic reference to the midline anterior border of the trachea is required for assessment, should bleeding occur, to help the surgeon plan whether the emergency operative approach should be a sternotomy to repair the right pulmonary artery, aorta, or innominate artery or a right thoracotomy to repair the azygous vein.

In this case, the dark (poorly oxygenated) blood and high-volume but low-pressure bleeding implied that either a pulmonary artery or azygous vein was the source. The azygous vein can easily be mistaken, as it courses from the posterior thorax to its junction with the back of the superior vena cava, for a back low right paratracheal node.

Bleeding from small veins can often be controlled with packing and pressure. Small bronchial arteries can often be controlled by hemoclips applied with a special long clip applier or cauterized with a special combined suction-Bovie catheter. Major arterial or venous hemorrhages require an open sternotomy or thoracotomy for direct suture repair. Injury to the pulmonary artery, if severe, may require formal cardiopulmonary bypass to decompress the pulmonary circuit and permit adequate visualization for repairing the vessel if proximal clamping of the right pulmonary artery is not possible. Arterial injury to the innominate artery or the aorta proper requires repair through a median sternotomy.

Other structures that can be injured during a mediastinoscopy include the left recurrent nerve, the esophagus, the trachea, and the right or left mainstem bronchi. The take-off of the right upper lobe bronchus, even as far distal as the right middle lobe bronchus, has been inadvertently injured during biopsies. Care must be taken when passing the scope in elderly patients with calcified vessels, because plaques can be dislodged and embolize into the cerebral circulation with pressure and upward leverage on the innominate artery.

Although mediastinoscopy is considered the gold standard for staging the mediastinum in patients with lung cancer who show enlarged mediastinal nodes (>1 cm) on CT scan, thoracoscopy and transtracheal or transthoracic aspiration of nodes have their proponents.

The intraoperative photograph shown (Figure 22-1) was taken during a radical resection of mediastinal nodes for recurrent thyroid carcinoma. The mediastinoscope has been positioned to demonstrate the plane of dissection during mediastinoscopy and the proximity of the scope with the major vascular structures.

CLINICAL POINTS TO REMEMBER

1. Thoracic residents and surgeons must have a detailed understanding of the three-dimensional anatomy of the mediastinum before performing mediastinoscopy.
2. Distortions related to malignancies or granulomatous disease must be taken into account before biopsy. A CT scan of the patient's chest should be available in the operating room for review before the procedure so that the particular details of a given patient's pathology and anatomy can be re-examined.
3. Deep aspiration of all lymph nodes must precede their biopsy.
4. Patients must be widely prepared and draped in case an emergency thoracotomy is required.

Figure 22-1 This mediastinoscope is in position during a radical dissection of mediastinal nodes.

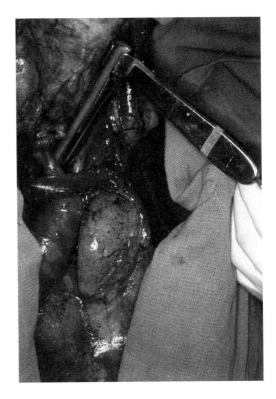

SELECTED READINGS

Gossot D, Toledo L, Fritsch S, Celerier M. Mediastinoscopy vs thoracoscopy for mediastinal biopsy. Results of a prospective nonrandomized study. Chest 1996;110:1328–1331.

Kirschner PA. Cervical mediastinoscopy. Chest Surg Clin North Am 1996;6:1–20.

23

The Man with a Slow Pulse and a Fast Cardiologist

Mr. Jones is a 76-year-old man who was recently evaluated for a syncopal episode. Evaluation on a 24-hour Holter monitor showed that he has a sick sinus syndrome. Elective placement of a ventricular demand inhibited pacemaker is recommended. Dr. Quickcard, a respected cardiologist who has placed hundreds of pacemakers during his career, arranges for outpatient placement of the pacemaker.

Mr. Jones is positioned on the fluoroscopy table, and his chest and deltopectoral groove are prepared and draped. Local anesthetic (1% lidocaine) is infiltrated, and the left subclavian vein is located and cannulated with a guidewire using the Seldinger technique. A vessel dilator and introducer are passed. A standard lead is passed through the introducer with a guidewire fashioned by Dr. Quickcard. Under fluoroscopic guidance, the lead is passed through the innominate venous bridge, into the superior vena cava, and through the right atrium and tricuspid valve. Several manipulations back and forth with different bendings of the guidewire are required before the lead is appropriately positioned and acceptable stimulation parameters are possible. Dr. Quickcard becomes a little frustrated because the procedure has taken twice as long as he had planned, and he is running behind. A subcutaneous pocket for the pacemaker is created, the lead is attached, and the skin is closed. The dressing is applied. Mr. Jones is transferred to the recovery area for a chest radiograph and 12-lead ECG. Dr. Quickcard completes the postoperative orders and returns to his busy clinic.

One hour later, the cardiologist receives an urgent page from the nurse in the recovery room. Mr. Jones is not feeling well; his systolic blood pressure is 70 mm Hg, and his heart rate is 100 bpm without paced beats. The chest radiograph demonstrates acceptable positioning of the lead in the apex of the right ventricle with clear lung markings. The cardiologist runs back to the recovery room and confirms the nurse's finding that Mr. Jones looks unwell and has what appear to be distended neck veins. A pulsus paradoxus of 20 mm Hg is found. An urgent cardiovascular surgical consult is obtained and, while the arrival of the surgeons is awaited, a portable echocardiogram demonstrates free fluid within the pericardial sac. A diagnosis of perforation of the right ventricle with cardiac tamponade is made. Mr. Jones is transported to the operating room immediately for repair of the injury. His recovery over the next few days is uneventful.

DISCUSSION

Iatrogenic injury to the heart can occur with a host of procedures and devices, including pacemaker leads, central lines, Swan-Ganz catheters, and right ventricular cardiac muscle biopsies used to monitor heart transplant graft rejection status. The thickness of the right-sided chambers (right atria and ventricle) is less than 1–3 mm. Conditions that result in chronic distention of these chambers (chronic obstructive pulmonary disease, cor pulmonale, pulmonic valvular disease) or place the chambers under higher than normal pressures can predispose to iatrogenic perforation.

Although perforation and tamponade can closely follow the procedure, perforation can also occur slowly with chronic use of indwelling catheters. Some perforations can be self-limited, but others can acutely bleed into the confined pericardial cavity and result in acute tamponade with as little as 75 ml of extravasated blood. The cardiac silhouette does not necessarily distend, as is seen in cases of chronic tamponade related to malignancies and uremia, in which several liters of fluid can accumulate over time with compensation by the heart. Clinical suspicion is needed to make the diagnosis. A pulsus paradoxus, which is the normal drop in systolic blood pressure that occurs with inspiration, is accentuated in tamponade and considered abnormal if the drop is greater than 10 mm Hg during normal respiration. Some practice is required to clinically note the changes in the Korotkoff sounds when manually measuring the blood pressure. A patient who is in the ICU with an indwelling arterial catheter can be diagnosed more easily by the variation in the pressure waves with the respiratory cycle.

The manner in which anesthesia is induced in these patients is critical, because many of them need protective sympathetic nervous system discharges to maintain blood pressure and increasing respiratory efforts to maintain venous return to the heart through the generated negative intrathoracic pressures. Induction of anesthesia with positive pressure ventilation and pharmacologic blunting of the effects of the catecholamine secretions can result in an immediate cardiovascular collapse and ventricular fibrillation. The surgeon must be in the room at the time of induction, preferably scrubbed, with the patient prepared and draped.

Occasionally, needle drainage of the pericardial sac before induction is required, or an initial decompression under local anesthesia through a subxiphoid approach with the patient awake may be necessary, if damage is severe. Pericardial windows for malignancy or uremia are usually created through a subxiphoid approach, with drainage of the pericardial fluid into the mediastinum where it is absorbed, or a small hole may be created in the central tendon of the diaphragm to permit drainage into the peritoneal cavity. A left thoracotomy or video-assisted technique is also performed in elective cases. Radical pericardiectomy for chronic tamponade, as seen in constrictive pericarditis from tuberculosis, requires either a sternotomy or a bilateral anterior thoracotomy with transverse sternotomy.

In this case of traumatic pericardial tamponade, a simple pledgetted suture in the right ventricular free wall corrected the problem, but a full sternotomy was required for the repair. Cardiopulmonary bypass was not required for this repair, but may be necessary for more complex traumatic injuries to the heart or in cases of decompression of chronically constricted sacs.

CLINICAL POINTS TO REMEMBER

1. Iatrogenic injury to the heart can occur in a host of procedures, including pacemaker insertion.
2. Although perforation and tamponade can closely follow the procedure, perforation can occur slowly with chronic use of indwelling catheters.
3. Mortality rates for patients with undiagnosed right ventricular perforation are high.

SELECTED READINGS

Gondi B, Nanda NC. Real-time, two-dimensional echocardiographic features of pacemaker perforation. Circulation 1981;64:97–106.

Gregoratos G, Cheitlin MD, Conill A, et al. ACC/AHA guidelines for implantation of cardiac pacemakers and antiarrhythmia devices: a report of the American College of Cardiology/American Heart Association Task Force on Practice Guidelines (Committee on Pacemaker Implantation). J Am Coll Cardiol 1998;31: 1175–1209.

Peters RW, Scheinman MM, Raskin S, Thomas AN. Unusual complications of epicardial pacemakers. Recurrent pericarditis, cardiac tamponade and pericardial constriction. Am J Cardiol 1980; 45:1088–1094.

24

The Heart Patient Who Induced Chest Pain in His Physician

Peter is a 44-year-old successful medical malpractice attorney for the plaintiff who presents to his physician with complaints of increasing fatigue during his golf game. In fact, he has added 10 strokes to his average and has started using a golf cart for every outing. He has a history of hypertension and moderate obesity, and a strong family history of coronary artery disease. Faced with this constellation of historical information and an unrevealing physical examination, Peter's physician recommends an exercise stress test as an initial diagnostic step. During stage II of a modified Bruce protocol, Peter exhibits 3 mm of flat ST segment depression in the anterior precordial ECG leads. He develops dyspnea and diaphoresis and is noted to have a nonsustained episode of wide-complex tachycardia. His physician, concerned about these events, calls a cardiology consultant, Dr. G, who arranges for an elective outpatient cardiac catheterization.

Peter, a curious and resourceful individual, spends most of the evening before his catheterization reading medical and legal treatises on catheterization, coronary artery disease, and their complications. Needless to say, he approaches his catheterization the next morning with some trepidation. He meticulously reads the preprinted informed consent form for catheterization and possible angioplasty. He also queries his cardiologist extensively regarding the doctor's experience in the cardiac catheterization laboratory. Dr. G's apprehension level rises as a result of his inquisitive patient.

While access is being obtained in the right groin, Peter complains of being warm and has an episode of bradycardia of 32 bpm. Dr. G has an episode of tachycardia with mild nausea. Peter responds to atropine and reassurance, and the procedure continues. Selective coronary arteriography reveals a single proximal left anterior descending coronary artery lesion of 80–90% stenosis that Dr. G judges to be amenable to balloon angioplasty. The balloon catheter is advanced across the lesion easily, and dilation is performed.

Shortly after removal of the balloon catheter, Peter complains of crushing substernal chest pain, and ST segment elevation is noted on the monitor. Closure of the left anterior descending coronary artery lesion is identified on arteriography with an appearance suggestive of acute thrombosis. During attempts to remediate the lesion, Peter develops sustained ventricular tachycardia with cardiorespiratory arrest. Dr. G institutes standard resuscitative techniques, including external chest compression, endotracheal intubation, epinephrine, and defibrillation, while summoning the cardiovascular surgical team for consideration of mechanical cardiovascular support and acute coronary bypass surgery. The code team arrives at the cardiac catheterization laboratory to assist Dr. G.

Peter, whose heart rhythm has deteriorated to ventricular fibrillation, is initially unresponsive to defibrillation attempts and intravenous epinephrine. An intra-aortic balloon pump is emergently placed, and, after administration of 100 mg of lidocaine and additional epinephrine, Peter is successfully defibrillated into sinus tachycardia. The surgical team transports the patient to the surgical suite, where an emergency bypass procedure is performed.

Fortunately, Peter survives his ordeal to initiate malpractice proceedings against Dr. G.

DISCUSSION

Angioplasty has been a remarkable addition to our armamentarium against coronary artery disease. When it is successful, substantial symptomatic improvement is seen. However, complications still arise during the procedure, including abrupt vessel closure, vessel dissections, and cardiac arrest.

Resuscitation from death is not an everyday event, but it is no longer a rarity. The evolution of CPR reflects a history of human error and human discovery, as does the evolution of medicine as a whole. Despite significant interest in exploring alternative methods, closed-chest compression remains the resuscitation technique used by most practitioners in the United States. Peter's cardiac arrest occurred in an ideal environment, with skilled practitioners in attendance.

The goal of resuscitation is restoration of normal or near-normal cardiopulmonary function without deterioration of other organ systems. The overall objective of CPR is to generate adequate blood flow of well-oxygenated blood to the heart and brain until more definitive therapy can be applied and spontaneous, effective circulation can be restored. During CPR, the dynamics of the chest compression process may play a major role in determining the outcome of the resuscitation effort. The best way to preserve neurologic function is early and effective restoration of cardiopulmonary function. If standard closed-chest compressions do not restore circulation promptly, cerebral survival is minimal. These observations have led investigators to seek new methods of resuscitation, with the hope of improving outcomes from cardiopulmonary arrest.

The basic life support guidelines established by the American Heart Association include a combination of external chest compression and ventilation. For resuscitative efforts and evaluation to be effective, the patient must be supine and on a firm, flat surface. Compressions are performed in the lower part of the sternum, 1.5 in. deep in the adult, at a rate of 80–100 compressions per minute. Arterial pressure during chest compression is maximal when the duration of compression is 50% of the compression-release cycle. Supplemental O_2 should be used as soon as possible. Rescue breathing delivers only 16–17% O_2 to the patient, ideally producing an alveolar O_2 tension of 80 mm Hg. Bag-valve devices, which consist of a self-inflating bag and nonrebreathing valve, may be used with a mask or endotracheal tube.

The trachea should be intubated by trained personnel as early in the resuscitative effort as is practical. Endotracheal intubation isolates the airway, keeps it patent, reduces the risk of aspiration, permits suctioning of the trachea, ensures delivery of a high concentration of O_2, and provides a route for the administration of certain drugs. This was promptly accomplished in Peter's case permitting high-concentration O_2 delivery.

Forward flow was previously believed to be caused by compression of the heart between the sternum and paraspinal structures, producing ejection of blood from the left ventricle into the systemic circulation (cardiac pump theory). Later studies have suggested that forward flow during CPR results from an increase in intrathoracic pressure that produces an arteriovenous pressure gradient in which the left ventricle acts as a passive conduit and not as a pump (thoracic pump theory). It is likely that both mechanisms result in forward blood flow. During cardiac arrest, properly performed chest compressions can produce systolic arterial blood pressure peaks of 60–80 mm Hg, but diastolic pressure remains low. Mean blood pressure in the carotid artery seldom exceeds 40 mm Hg. Cardiac output resulting from chest compressions is only one-fourth to one-third of normal.

A number of simple and not-so-simple mechanical devices have been developed to aid resuscitation efforts. The simplest of these devices, the cardiac press, is a hinge (manually operated) that provides some mechanical advantage for the rescuer performing chest compressions. This device may help ensure standard position in CPR technique and eliminate some rescuer fatigue. It can be applied relatively quickly, but may move around the chest, so its position must be monitored carefully.

Pneumatically powered mechanical resuscitators programmed to the American Heart Association guidelines are available. Their principal advantage is their ability to free a single trained person to participate in the delivery of advanced cardiac life support when the number of rescuers is limited. This mechanical device permits prolonged resuscitative efforts. Rapid cyclical inflation of a vest surrounding the chest (pressure level 200–250 mm Hg), has been described by Halperin and coworkers to improve coronary blood flow in a canine cardiac arrest model. However, Swenson and coauthors found that simultaneous ventilation and pneumatic vest compression adversely affected coronary perfusion.

As in Peter's case, intra-aortic balloon pumps and percutaneous cardiopulmonary bypass have occasionally been used in patients after a cardiac arrest. However, the widespread application of these techniques is problematic because the required equipment is cumbersome, difficult to use, and not easily available.

CLINICAL POINTS TO REMEMBER

1. Maximal resuscitation is likely to occur after skillful application of proper CPR techniques.
2. Compression rates and depths should follow the American Heart Association standards.
3. Defibrillation is the single most important component of advanced cardiac life support.

4. Endotracheal intubation with 100% O_2 administration should be an early priority.
5. Coronary blood flow and, therefore, aortic diastolic pressure are important determinants of resuscitability.

SELECTED READINGS

Ambrose JA, Almeida OD, Sharma SK, et al. Angiographic evolution of intracoronary thrombus and dissection following percutaneous transluminal coronary angioplasty (the Thrombolysis and Angioplasty in Unstable Angina [TAUSA] trial). Am J Cardiol 1997;79:559–563.

Fromm RE, Varon J, Stahmer SA. Techniques in cardiopulmonary resuscitation: past, present and future. Hosp Physician 1994;30(7):10–13, 30.

Marti V, Martin V, Garcia J, et al. Significance of angiographic coronary dissection after cutting balloon angioplasty. Am J Cardiol 1998;81: 1349–1352.

Varon J, Fromm RE. Cardiopulmonary resuscitation: new and controversial techniques. Postgrad Med 1993;93:235–242.

Varon J, Marik PE, Fromm RE. Cardiopulmonary resuscitation: a review for clinicians. Resuscitation 1998;36:133–145.

Varon J, Sternbach GL. Cardiopulmonary resuscitation: lessons from the past. J Emerg Med 1991;9:503–507.

Voigtländer T, Rupprecht HJ, Scharhag J, et al. Intravascular ultrasound detected classification of coronary lesions as a predictor of dissections after balloon angioplasty. Int J Card Imaging 1996;12:179–183.

25

The College Freshman with Warm Hands but Cold Feet

Edwin is a handsome, apparently healthy young freshman at Rice University, born and raised in the small town of Paris, Texas. He is majoring in biology and American history. He has always been outgoing and popular with girls and has always been kidded about his very warm hands and ice-cold feet.

During the second week of his first term, he is taking notes in a crowded classroom and is surprised to notice the sudden onset of brisk epistaxis. He had one previous major nosebleed during the past 6 months that responded to prolonged pressure on the nasal septum, which he attributed to the drying effects of his air conditioner at home. During the present episode, he quickly excuses himself, leaves the classroom, and goes to the rest room, but persistent pressure does not control the hemorrhage. Another student happens to come into the washroom at this moment and notices his predicament. The campus police are called, and they quickly rush him to a Texas Medical Center Hospital.

On arrival at the ED, the epistaxis has abated. Edwin had planned to return to class without being evaluated, but the triage nurse has taken his initial blood pressure reading and discovered severe systolic hypertension of 260/90 mm Hg. The emergency physician confirms this reading, checks the contralateral arm, and finds a similar pressure reading at the elbow.

On closer examination, Edwin is found to have prominent pulsations in the suprasternal notch and a systolic murmur that radiates to his back in the interscapular region. His legs are cold, and palpating either femoral pulse is difficult. ECG is performed and reveals left ventricular hypertrophy. An esophageal contrast radiograph is taken (Figure 25-1). A tentative diagnosis of aortic coarctation is made. An echocardiogram does not demonstrate any associated cardiac abnormalities, and the aor-

tic valve is normal. An arteriogram is obtained and primary
repair of the lesion recommended.

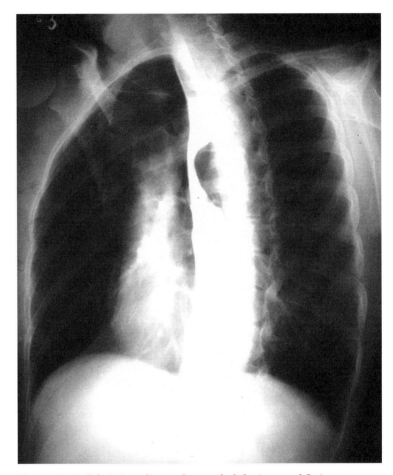

Figure 25-1 Edwin's radiograph revealed the inverted 3 sign.

DISCUSSION

Coarctation of the aorta is a narrowing of the aorta where the distal arch ends and the proximal descending aorta begins, in the region of the ductus arteriosus. Coarctations have been described both before and after the entrance of the ductus arteriosus. Decreased left-sided blood flow in utero that results in less blood flowing through the aortic isthmus leads to underdevelopment of this area and possibly to a preductal coarctation.

Aortic stenosis, a bicuspid aortic valve, mitral stenosis, and hypoplastic left heart syndrome can be associated with this infantile type of preductal coarctation. Often children with this condition are extremely ill and quickly decompensate when the ductus starts to close shortly after birth. They develop mottling of their abdomen and legs and severe acidosis. More than half of all children with coarctation present with symptoms within the first few months of life.

A second type of coarctation, sometimes known as *adult-type coarctation* (although this is a misnomer, because it occurs in children as well), is described as an intraluminal shelf-like narrowing from thickening of the aortic media that occurs just beyond and distal to the entrance of the ductus arteriosus. Depending on the degree to which the aorta has narrowed, this can result in severe congestive heart failure in infants or in a delayed diagnosis, as it did in Edwin. With time, a significant arterial collateral circulation develops. Branches from the subclavian and axillary arteries, including the internal mammary, thyrocervical, and costocervical trunks and the lateral thoracic arteries, can all feed intercostal vessels that carry blood retrograde into the distal thoracic aorta below the aortic narrowing. Enlarged intercostal arteries can result in rib notching on plain chest radiographs.

A variety of surgical techniques have been used to treat coarctation when it presents in infancy, including primary end-to-end anastomosis with resection of the narrowing and a turn-down subclavian flap technique that is preferred by many surgeons because it permits growth of the aorta over time, with less need to reoperate for restenosis. Dissolving monofilament sutures that permit growth of the arteriotomy closure are preferred. Many children require repair of associated intracardiac defects, including ventricular septal defects, patent ductus arteriosus, and aortic and mitral valvular lesions. Complete repair of all defects in neonates through an anterior sternotomy approach has been described; the mobility of neonatal tissues permits an approach that is not possible in older children. Symptomatic infants with coarctations who are not diagnosed or not treated surgically have a mortality rate close to 90%.

As in Edwin's case, less severe forms of coarctation can remain asymptomatic for many years, even into young adulthood. The physical examination usually points to the diagnosis by revealing that femoral pulses are absent or delayed when compared to the upper extremities. Adults usually die as a result of the complications of prolonged hypertension. The hypertension is thought to have a renal origin.

Epistaxis was a fortuitous early warning of Edwin's uncontrolled hypertension. Adults can die of aortic dissection or rupture or of intracranial hemorrhage. Cardiac failure can develop in adults as it can in infants, but in adults it is a late sign of a chronically afterloaded left ventricle. Such patients are also susceptible to infective endarteritis related to the turbulent flow in the region of the coarctation; this can affect the aortic valve (often bicuspid) or prompt the development of a mycotic aneurysm in the poststenotic dilated portion of the aorta.

Surgery in the adult usually entails a posterolateral thoracotomy through the fourth intercostal space. This is often an extremely tedious dissection because of the significant collaterals that develop around the chest wall. Special care is taken not to injure the enlarged posterior intercostal arteries, which can be extremely friable and difficult to control. The recurrent laryngeal nerve is identified and preserved as it courses around the ligamentum arteriosus.

The anesthesiologist must be extremely vigilant about blood pressure control with aortic clamping and unclamping. Usually a primary end-to-end anastomosis is possible after resection of the narrowed segment; however, short interposition grafts are occasionally required and subclavian flaps and various aortoplasty techniques have been used. Paradoxical hypertension and severe abdominal pain are seen postoperatively in some patients, but usually they resolve when treated symptomatically.

The surgical mortality in experienced medical centers is low for repairs in infants and adults (less than 1%). The occurrence of persistent postoperative hypertension is inversely related to the age of repair: rare in infants and up to 50% in adults.

CLINICAL POINTS TO REMEMBER

1. Aortic coarctation can remain asymptomatic for many years, even into young adulthood.
2. Enlarged intercostal arteries can result in rib notching on plain chest radiographs.
3. The physical examination usually points to the diagnosis by revealing that femoral pulses are absent or delayed when compared to the upper extremities. Adults usually die as a result of the complications of prolonged hypertension.
4. The overall mortality rate for repairs of aortic coarctation is less than 1%.

5. The occurrence of persistent postoperative hypertension is inversely related to the age of repair: rare in infants and up to 50% in adults.

SELECTED READINGS

Hirooka K, Fraser CD Jr. One-stage neonatal repair of complex aortic arch obstruction or interruption. Recent experience at Texas Children's Hospital. Tex Heart Inst J 1997;24:317–321.

Ing FF, Starc TJ, Griffiths SP, Gersony WM. Early diagnosis of coarctation of the aorta in children: a continuing dilemma. Pediatrics 1996;98:378–382.

Pfammatter JP, Ziemer G, Kaulitz R, et al. Isolated aortic coarctation in neonates and infants: results of resection and end-to-end anastomosis. Ann Thorac Surg 1996;62:778–782.

Wells WJ, Prendergast TW, Berdjis F, et al. Repair of coarctation of the aorta in adults: the fate of systolic hypertension. Ann Thorac Surg 1996;61:1168–1171.

Wiest DB, Garner SS, Uber WE, Sade RM. Esmolol for the management of pediatric hypertension after cardiac operations. J Thorac Cardiovasc Surg 1998;115:890–897.

26

The Opera Singer with a Hoarse Voice

Mary, a 46-year-old nonsmoker, is a well-known soprano who has been with the Houston Opera for more than 4 years. She has been practicing extremely hard over the past 3 months for her upcoming presentation of Queen of the Night in *The Magic Flute*, for which the company has scheduled a 6-month, 35-city tour that will include major European centers.

During a recital, Mary is unable to reach some high notes. She sees her primary care physician, who performs an indirect laryngoscopy in the office with a mirror and believes that the left vocal cord is erythematous and possibly has a polyp. This is thought to be caused by voice strain, and a period of voice rest is prescribed. Some transient improvement occurs, but on returning to singing 2 weeks later, Mary is again unable to perform, and she develops a dry cough and some hoarseness of her voice during normal conversation.

Mary returns to her primary care physician, who has recently purchased a fiberoptic laryngoscope for his office. While the clinician is trying to diagnose Mary's problem with his new instrument, several attempts at direct laryngoscopy are made. Mary suddenly develops stridor and significant dyspnea, and her physician activates emergency medical services by calling 911. On arriving at the physician's office, the paramedics promptly intubate Mary and transport her to the local hospital, where she is admitted to the ICU with a diagnosis of iatrogenic upper airway obstruction.

Within 24 hours of admission to the ICU, Mary is extubated and evaluated by the otolaryngology services, who find a paralysis of her left vocal cord without any mucosal or vocal cord lesions. A chest radiograph ordered on admission reveals left upper lobe density and an abnormal mediastinal shadow. A CT scan of the chest is obtained (Figure 26-1). Further testing reveals the cause of her hoarseness to be a left upper lobe malignancy with bulky mediastinal adenopathy.

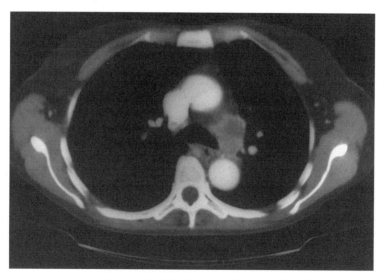

Figure 26-1   A bulky mediastinal aortopulmonary lymph node from the left upper lobe lung cancer caused left recurrent nerve paralysis.

DISCUSSION

Voice hoarseness can result from a variety of causes, including inflammation of the larynx as part of viral upper respiratory tract infections and intrinsic vocal cord or laryngeal pathology such as polyps or invasive malignancies.

A paretic or paralyzed cord without intrinsic laryngeal pathology, as is demonstrated in this case, usually is the result of displacement, compression, or direct involvement of the recurrent laryngeal nerve along its course by a variety of lesions, including vascular aneurysms and benign and malignant tumors of the head, neck, and thoracic cavity. This can involve the vagus nerve proper, or it may involve the recurrent nerve from its take-off from the vagus in the left hemithorax as it swings around the ligamentum arteriosum, courses along the left tracheoesophageal groove, and penetrates the cricothyroid membrane. The right recurrent nerve courses around the right subclavian artery and takes a more acute angle back to the larynx.

The CT scan in this case demonstrated a left upper lobe lung cancer with extensive mediastinal lymphadenopathy involving the aortopulmonary window. Although this patient was young and a nonsmoker, nearly 5% of patients with lung cancer do not have a history of smoking exposure. Histologic diagnosis can be made easily through transthoracic needle aspiration of the aortopulmonary lymph node or through bronchoscopy and fluoroscopically guided biopsy of the primary lesion. In a patient with a suspected lymphoma (who may have B symptoms with bulky mediastinal nodes), a larger biopsy is required for histologic subtyping. A mediastinotomy anteriorly through the second or third intercostal space (the Chamberlain procedure) or a video-assisted thoracoscopic biopsy is often required.

A patient with lung cancer who presents with a hoarse voice is usually inoperable and should be considered for chemotherapy and radiation therapy protocols once the histologic subtype of the lung cancer is confirmed (small cell vs. non–small cell) and the metastatic staging is complete. The median survival of patients presenting with stage III disease is 18 months. With treatment, the voice hoarseness may improve, although hoarseness in patients with malignancies is usually related to direct invasion rather than compression of the nerve. Because the recurrent nerve also controls the function of the inferior constrictors of the pharynx, patients may be susceptible to silent aspiration and pneumonia. The remaining functioning cord partially compensates for a paralyzed cord. In those patients whose hoarseness significantly affects quality of life by preventing effective communication, techniques are available to improve voice quality. These include medialization of the paralyzed cord and Teflon or autologous fat injection of the paretic cord. These techniques can improve quality of life for these patients, although sadly this patient's singing career was over as a result of the unresectable squamous cell lung carcinoma.

CLINICAL POINTS TO REMEMBER

1. Voice hoarseness can result from a variety of causes, including invasive malignancies.
2. A paretic or paralyzed cord without intrinsic laryngeal pathology usually is a result of displacement, compression, or direct involvement of the recurrent laryngeal nerve along its course.
3. A patient with lung cancer who presents with a hoarse voice is usually inoperable.

SELECTED READINGS

Berke GS, Kevorkian KF. The diagnosis and management of hoarseness. Compr Ther 1996;22: 251–255.

MacKenzie K. Diagnosis and treatment of hoarseness. Practitioner 1994;238:474–478.

Rosen CA, Anderson D, Murry T. Evaluating hoarseness: keeping your patient's voice healthy. Am Fam Physician 1998;57:2775–2782.

27

A Third-Year Anesthesia Resident Armed with a Double-Lumen Tube

Sam is starting the third year of his anesthesia residency and is rotating through the thoracic service. He is preparing to induce a 56-year-old, 80-kg man, once a heavy smoker, who is scheduled to undergo a left upper lobectomy for a newly discovered spiculated tumor that measures 4 cm in diameter (stage T2). The patient's pulmonary function tests demonstrate an FEV_1 that is 83% of the predicted volume. The CT scan demonstrates no evidence of enlarged mediastinal nodes, so a mediastinoscopy is not planned.

The endobronchial anatomy is assessed using a flexible adult bronchoscope passed through a laryngeal mask airway; the bronchoscope is initially used to secure the airway. After this, a double-lumen tube is placed. At the time of the placement of the double-lumen tube, the larynx appears very anterior, which necessitates several attempts to visualize the vocal cords. The lubricated double-lumen tube (39 Fr) is passed through the cords, but this requires some pressure. Once through the cords, the tube is rotated counterclockwise to seat the left-sided bronchial blocker in the left mainstem bronchus. The end-tidal CO_2 monitor confirms a good waveform. The bronchial balloon is inflated, and the position of the double-lumen tube is checked by clinical examination (sequential clamping of each lumen of the double-lumen tube) and by endoscopic verification using a small flexible fiberoptic bronchoscope. The blue balloon of the bronchial blocker can be well visualized when properly in the left mainstem bronchus with the proximal margin of the balloon at the level of the main carina. The tube is taped in place.

A central venous right-sided internal jugular line and a right radial arterial line for continuous blood pressure monitoring are placed uneventfully. Preparations are made to roll the patient into a right lateral decubitus position in readiness for the left thoracotomy. The bronchial blocker in the left mainstem bronchus is deflated before rolling the patient to avoid injury to the membranous portion of the left mainstem bronchus by the balloon.

While the patient is being secured in the right lateral decubitus position, peak airway pressures are noted to suddenly elevate into the range of 60 cm H_2O; the patient becomes hypotensive to 70 mm Hg and is progressively more bradycardic to approximately 40 bpm. He is quickly moved into a supine position. Auscultation of the chest demonstrates significantly decreased breath sounds over the right hemithorax. A pneumothorax secondary to the placement of the central line is suspected, and a 14-gauge angiocatheter is placed through the second intercostal space in the midclavicular line. Immediately, air under pressure is encountered, and the diagnosis of a tension pneumothorax is confirmed. The patient's blood pressure transiently improves.

A 28-Fr chest tube is placed through the fifth intercostal space and connected to an underwater seal. A significant air leak is noted, far greater than expected from a simple needle-stick during central line placement. A portable chest radiograph is performed and demonstrates a persistent airspace and incomplete expansion of the right lung. The chest tube is connected to suction, and the air leak gets worse. Suction is stopped as ventilation fails.

At this point, a small amount of subcutaneous emphysema is noted in the supraclavicular notch. An injury to the tracheobronchial tree secondary to traumatic intubation is suspected. The small bronchoscope is advanced through the bronchial lumen of the double-lumen tube, and the tube is slowly withdrawn with both balloons deflated. As the tube is withdrawn into the main trachea, a midline linear 1.5-cm tear of the membranous trachea is noted, with the distal portion of the tear 2 cm cephalad to the main carina. Preparations are made for an emergency repair of the iatrogenic injury.

DISCUSSION

The adult trachea is fairly uniform in size throughout its length; it is composed of 1,620 hyaline cartilage rings connected to each other by connective and elastic tissues that permit some lengthening and flexion of the trachea over its 10-cm length. The membranous portion posteriorly is a continuation of the anterior fibrous tissue combined with smooth muscle lined by epithelium and glands. It is distensible and permits some increase in the diameter of the trachea, depending on the physiologic needs (e.g., deep inspiration and coughing).

In an anesthetized patient, the membranous trachea can be torn. As it is stretched between relatively fixed cartilaginous rings posteriorly, it is subject to injury, much as the tightly stretched skin of a snare drum may be highly resistant to pressure distributed over a broad surface area but can easily tear should a sharp object be pushed along the surface. Special care must be taken in introducing endotracheal tubes with stylets to ensure that a stylet does not pass the tip of the tube, and in introducing oversized endotracheal tubes that may stretch the trachea to the point of breaking. Other airway manipulations, such as rigid bronchoscopy and inadvertent passage of a nasogastric tube into the airway, can result in upper airway injury.

Iatrogenic injury to the tracheobronchial tree, like injuries from blunt or sharp trauma, can be initially overlooked or misinterpreted. A finding of a significant air leak when the lung cannot be fully inflated with one or two chest tubes is usually indicative of a major central airway injury. If the injury does not communicate with the pleural space, peribronchial or peritracheal tissues can seal the leak, and delayed recognition through airway stricture development, distal pulmonary infections, or bronchiectasis results. If the distal lung is not infected, primary repair of the injury is usually possible without loss of functional lung tissue. If the distal lung tissue is infected or fibrotic, resection may be required.

Diagnosis of airway injury is much easier when there is free communication with the pleural space. In this case, the injury presented with a tension pneumothorax. Repair of such injuries requires close communication between the anesthesiologist and the thoracic surgeon. Selection of ventilating tubes that permit ventilation of one or both lungs, depending on the location of the injury, and dissection and primary repair of the injury must be discussed in great detail. Should complete transection of an airway be encountered, jet ventilation techniques or the use of two ventilators with intermittent ventilation across the operating table may be required.

Most injuries of the cervical trachea can be approached through a collar neck incision. Injuries of the lower trachea and proximal left mainstem bronchus are approached through a right posterolateral thoracotomy through the fourth or fifth intercostal space. Distal left mainstem injuries are approached through a left thoracotomy. Absorbable suture material is used in most repairs, instead of monofilament sutures that can lead to granulation tissue formation and the need for resection, laser therapy, or stenting should stricturing develop.

Circumferential dissection of the trachea should be avoided to minimize the devascularization of the airway. The recurrent nerves, which course in the tracheoesophageal groove, must be identified and preserved. Autologous tissue is used to buttress the repair; in this case, an intercostal muscle pedicle was ideal. Thymic tissue, pericardium, and pleura are excellent for coverage when the repair is in the chest, and strap muscles and the sternocleidomastoid muscles are useful for repairs in the neck. Extubation in such cases should be performed as soon after the repair as possible to avoid positive pressure ventilation on the repair and endotracheal cuff injury near the repair. Tracheostomies should also be avoided. Special attention is given to controlling pain to assist in pulmonary toilet postoperatively, and directed bronchoscopic suctioning is used liberally in patients who have difficulty clearing their secretions.

CLINICAL POINTS TO REMEMBER

1. In an anesthetized patient, the membranous trachea can be torn.
2. Diagnosis of airway injury is much easier when there is free communication with the pleural space.
3. Injury to the tracheobronchial tree can be initially overlooked or misinterpreted.
4. Most injuries of the cervical trachea can be approached through a collar neck incision. Injuries of the lower trachea and proximal left mainstem bronchus are approached through a right posterolateral thoracotomy through the fourth or fifth intercostal space. Distal left mainstem injuries are approached through a left thoracotomy.

SELECTED READINGS

Devitt JH, Boulanger BR. Lower airway injuries and anaesthesia. Can J Anaesth 1996;43:148–159.

Lobato EB, Risley WP III, Stoltzfus DP. Intraoperative management of distal tracheal rupture with selective bronchial intubation. Clin Anesth 1997;9:155–158.

Massard G, Rouge C, Dabbagh A, et al. Tracheobronchial lacerations after intubation and tracheostomy. Ann Thorac Surg 1996;61: 1483–1487.

Ratzenhofer-Komenda B, Prause G, Offner A, et al. Tracheal disruption and pneumothorax as intraoperative complications. Acta Anaesthesiol Scand 1997;111(Suppl):314–317.

van Klarenbosch J, Meyer J, de Lange JJ. Tracheal rupture after tracheal intubation. Br J Anaesth 1994;73:550–551.

Yamazaki M, Sasaki R, Masuda A, Ito Y. Anesthetic management of complete tracheal disruption using percutaneous cardiopulmonary support system. Anesth Analg 1998;86:998–1000.

28
Gone Fishing

Ralph is a 48-year-old man from Lake Charles, Louisiana, who has a long history of hypertension and adult-onset diabetes mellitus. Ralph was initially admitted to the local community hospital with a diagnosis of pulmonary edema and subsequent respiratory failure. Despite placement of a pulmonary artery catheter and several days of diuresis, he was unable to be weaned from mechanical ventilation and had to be transferred for further management.

On arriving at our hospital, Ralph is intubated and on assisted mechanical ventilation. His blood pressure is elevated at 170/92 mm Hg, and his heart rate is 108 bpm. He is afebrile, rales and rhonchi are heard in both lung fields, and an S_4 gallop sound is also audible. A right subclavian pulmonary artery catheter is noted. The device was placed without the benefit of an introducer and had been pulled back to the central venous pressure position before Ralph was transferred. This line is the only IV access in place. The puncture site looks clean, and the line is secured with tape and a dressing.

After initial assessment, the house officers feel that further diuresis and afterload reduction will benefit Ralph, and that a triple-lumen catheter should replace the pulmonary artery catheter. Rather than subject Ralph to a new central venous puncture, the critical care fellow on call instructs the resident to change the line using a guidewire. The resident, while attempting to replace the line, realizes that the available guidewire is too short to divert any of the lumens of the pulmonary artery catheter. As a resourceful recent graduate, the resident elects to cut the pulmonary artery catheter near the point at which it enters the skin, cannulating one of the lumens with the guidewire and, thus, easily replacing the line. Unfortunately, while he is attempting to cannulate the transected catheter, the pulmonary artery catheter slips through his fingers and disappears beyond the puncture site. A short run of ventricular tachycardia is noted on the monitor and the resident is confident that it actually reflects "his own heart beat." The senior attending physician in the ICU is called at once, and a chest radiograph is obtained that reveals a catheter fragment lodged in the right ventricle. The patient is taken to the cardiac catheterization laboratory for retrieval of the fragment.

DISCUSSION

Almost any type of catheter, guidewire, or transvenous device may embolize to the central venous circulation. Improvements in catheter design and techniques have reduced the risk of this potentially lethal complication, but the increasing frequency of the use of these devices has led to increased risk.

Polyethylene central venous catheters are the devices most commonly reported to embolize. However, embolization of guidewires, pacemaker catheters, and ventricular venous shunt catheters has also been reported. Embolization of catheter fragments or guidewires to the heart or central circulation is not a trivial event. Many complications have been reported, including endocarditis, abscess, sepsis, vascular or cardiac perforation, dysrhythmias, and sudden death; mortality has been estimated at 25–50%.

When emboli do occur, efforts should be made to remove them in almost all cases, preferably using transvascular procedures. In this particular case, the lack of judgment on the part of the house officer led to inadvertent embolization of the distal portion of the pulmonary artery catheter. More commonly, piercing or cutting of polyethylene tubing by the sharp bevel of the needle in through-the-needle systems leads to embolization. Other potential mechanisms include manufacturing defects and improper or careless handling of catheters.

Before any attempt at retrieval, the catheter fragment should be localized, with particular attention to the proximal and distal tip of the catheter to determine whether these are free. The most common sites for catheter emboli are the superior vena cava, right atrium, right ventricle, internal jugular vein, subclavian vein, hepatic vein, inferior vena cava, pulmonary artery, and thoracic descending aorta. Transvascular techniques for removal are effective in 90% of embolism cases and are the procedures of choice. Transvascular retrieval is best performed in a room equipped with standard radiographic and fluoroscopic equipment; a cardiac catheterization suite is ideally equipped. Many different devices have been used to remove emboli, including loop-snare devices, helical baskets, and grasping forceps. Choice of device depends on the preferences of the operator and the specific characteristics and location of the embolus.

CLINICAL POINTS TO REMEMBER

1. Any type of catheter, guidewire, or transvenous device may embolize to the central venous circulation.
2. The most common sites for catheter emboli are the superior vena cava, right atrium, right ventricle, internal jugular vein, subclavian vein, hepatic vein, inferior vena cava, pulmonary artery, and thoracic descending aorta.
3. When emboli do occur, efforts should be made to remove them in almost all cases, preferably using transvascular procedures.
4. Transvascular retrieval is best performed in a room equipped with standard radiographic and fluoroscopic equipment; a cardiac catheterization suite is ideally equipped.

SELECTED READINGS

Bashour TT, Banks T, Cheng TO. Retrieval of lost catheters by a myocardial catheter biopsy device. Chest 1974;66:395–396.

Kaushik VS, Ong SH. Non-surgical retrieval of intracardiac foreign body: use of Berens pacing electrode. Am Heart J 1983;105:868–870.

Tilkian AG, Daily EK. Transluminal Catheter Extraction and Resolution of Intracardiac Catheter Knots. In AG Tilkian, EK Daily (eds), Cardiovascular Procedures. Diagnostic Techniques and Therapeutic Procedures. St. Louis: Mosby, 1986;390–406.

29

What Goes Down Often Comes Up

Amer is a 70-year-old man who presented to the hospital with complaints of abdominal pain, nausea, vomiting, and low grade fever. His past medical history is pertinent for hypertension, diabetes mellitus, and hypothyroidism, all of which appear to be poorly controlled. On review of systems, Amer also relates that he has experienced a decrease in his urinary stream and that the abdominal discomfort has been associated with dysuria. Physical examination reveals that Amer is febrile to 40°C. His skin turgor is poor, and his mucous membranes are dry. An S_4 gallop sound is heard on auscultation of the chest, and the point of maximal intensity is displaced to the anterior axillary line. Few bowel sounds are heard during abdominal examination. No tenderness, guarding, or rebound is demonstrated. A rectal examination reveals a tender, boggy prostate.

Amer's white blood cell count is 15,700 cells/ml with 75% polymorphonuclear leukocytes and 12% band forms. Urinalysis demonstrates pyuria with bacteriuria and a dipstick positive for protein, glucose, and blood.

Amer is initially admitted to the floor but subsequently deteriorates and displays altered mental status, hypotension, worsening fever, and dyspnea. He is transferred to the ICU, where endotracheal intubation with assisted mechanical ventilation is instituted. Blood cultures obtained on admission grow *Escherichia coli*, and his antimicrobial regimen is appropriately adjusted. His condition stabilizes, and a nasoduodenal tube is placed by Nurse Allie for enteral feedings.

Dr. Jones is asked to examine Amer because increasing sputum production and high peak airway pressures are noted on the ventilator from the time of Amer's arrival at the ICU. As part of the evaluation, Dr. Jones requests a chest radiograph (Figure 29-1) but is called away to see another patient in a different floor before he can review it. Two hours later, Nurse Allie again pages Dr. Jones because of Amer's worsening hypoxemia and increased airway pressures. Dr. Jones obtains the previously performed chest radiograph and makes a diagnosis of nasoduodenal tube misplacement in the lung. He promptly removes the nasoduodenal tube from Amer's lung. Amer's condition stabilizes and over several days gradually improves.

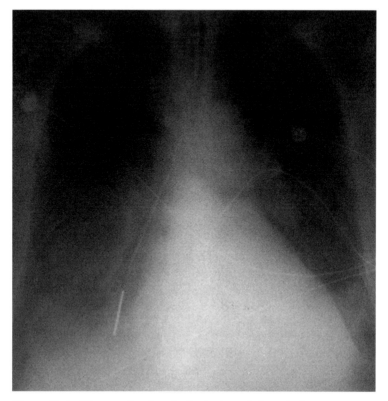

Figure 29-1 The nasoduodenal tube in Amer's lung is shown.

DISCUSSION

Nasoenteral tube placement is a common procedure in the ICU; in most instances it is delegated to the nursing service. Because most patients tolerate this procedure without complication, many physicians do not recognize the potential for adverse consequences.

In Amer's case, an inadvertent bronchial intubation was not recognized, and instillation of enteral feedings into the lung occurred. Because of these rare but serious consequences, many institutions require confirmation of tube placement by radiography before the tube is used for feeding.

To avoid misplacement, the patient should be placed in a left lateral decubitus position (if possible) when a nasoduodenal tube is placed using the bedside method. The patient's nostril is lubricated with generic lubricant or 2% viscous lidocaine, and an 8- to 10-Fr small-bore feeding tube (containing a wire stylet) is inserted into the nostril and gently advanced through the nasopharynx into the esophagus and the stomach. If resistance is met, a decrease in oxygen saturation is noted, or the patient coughs or becomes agitated, the tube should be pulled back into the nasopharynx and reinserted into the stomach. Changing the position of the patient's neck by flexing or extending it slightly before reattempting insertion can be helpful. To confirm the position of the tube in the stomach, auscultation of the abdomen and aspiration of the gastric contents (pH of 2–5, unless the patient is on an H_2 blocker) are performed.

Once the tube's position in the stomach is confirmed, the wire stylet is removed and a 45-degree bend is made approximately 1 in. from the distal end of the wire. The wire stylet is gently reinserted—it should not meet resistance—and the tube is slowly advanced while being rotated clockwise. Tube position must be checked every 10–15 cm; auscultation will reveal higher-pitched sounds when the tube is in the pylorus and proximal small bowel. Bile may be aspirated from the tube when it enters the small bowel (bile/small bowel secretions have a pH of 6–7). An abdominal x-ray can confirm small bowel location; it may not be cost-effective, but it can help avoid feeding into a lung.

If bedside placement is not possible, the feeding tube should be placed in the small intestine using endoscopy or fluoroscopy. In patients undergoing abdominal surgery, the tube should be placed during surgery under direct visualization. In these patients, the anesthesiologist is usually the one to insert the tube into the stomach; the surgeon locates the tube and directs it into duodenum or jejunum. This method eliminates the need for confirmatory x-rays and allows immediate feeding on the patient's admission to the ICU. Feeding tubes may also be placed in the small bowel using a gastrostomy or jejunostomy.

CLINICAL POINTS TO REMEMBER

1. Inadvertent bronchial intubation of nasoenteral tubes is a rare but well-documented complication of this procedure.
2. To confirm the position of the tube in the stomach, auscultation of the abdomen and aspiration of the gastric contents are performed.
3. Tubes placed in the stomach rarely (5–15% of the time) migrate spontaneously into the small bowel in critically ill patients.

SELECTED READINGS

Harrison AM, Clay B, Grant MJ, et al. Nonradiographic assessment of enteral feeding tube position. Crit Care Med 1997;25:2055–2059.

Scholten DJ, Wood TL, Thompson DR. Pneumothorax from nasoenteric feeding tube insertion. A report of five cases. Am Surg 1986;52:381–385.

Woodall BH, Winfield DF, Bisset GS. Inadvertent tracheobronchial placement of feeding tubes. Radiology 1987;165:727–729.

Zaloga GP. Bedside method for placing small bowel feeding tubes in critically ill patients. Chest 1991;100:1643–1646.

30

The Cocaine Abuser with Not Enough Blood and Too Much Phosphate

George, a 27-year-old man, is brought to the ED by paramedics after sustaining a stab wound to his left hemithorax while trying to buy cocaine from a local supplier. Apparently, he was trying to get a better deal, and his supplier got upset and attacked him with a large machete. George was able to run away, but after a few feet, he collapsed. On arriving at the scene, paramedics reported a large volume of blood on the floor. An IV line was started, and George was rapidly transported to the ED.

His initial physical examination reveals systolic blood pressure of 50 mm Hg, a pulse of 160 bpm, a respiratory rate of 40 breaths per minute (the Kussmaul pattern), and a temperature of 36.2°C. George is conscious but not responsive to verbal stimuli. His skin is pale and diaphoretic. The rest of the physical examination is unremarkable, except for a deep 6-cm transverse laceration across the left hemithorax between the fourth and sixth intercostal spaces at the midaxillary line that is bleeding briskly and requires the application of continued pressure. An audible air leak is heard by the physician taking care of George.

George is initially resuscitated with rapid IV infusion of 4 liters of lactated Ringer's solution, a tube thoracostomy, and endotracheal intubation, which resulted in blood pressure of 100/37 mm Hg and a pulse of 110 bpm. His initial laboratory data are remarkable for a white blood cell count of 11,000 cells/μl, hemoglobin of 11.1 gm/dl, and hematocrit of 33.6%. Arterial blood gases while the patient is on 100% O_2 reveal pH of 6.94, PCO_2 of 45 mm Hg, and PO_2 of 147 mm Hg. A chest radiograph reveals a left hydropneumothorax.

George is taken immediately to the operating room, where bleeding is controlled. He is transferred to the surgical ICU. Shortly thereafter, George becomes hypotensive again. A repeat hematocrit is 25%. No further clinical bleeding is noted. Packed red blood cells, 2U, are administered, and 35 minutes after the infusion starts, his blood pressure is 129/48 mm Hg and his pulse is 104 bpm. One ampule of sodium bicarbonate is administered intravenously. An echocardiogram reveals normal left ventricular function and no evidence of pericardial effusion.

George experiences no further hypotensive episodes. Repeat arterial blood gases after fluid resuscitation show a pH of 7.29, P_{CO_2} of 29 mm Hg, and P_{O_2} of 130 mm Hg. Analysis of blood drawn on initiation of treatment in the ED (and before the administration of red blood cells) reveals glucose of 203 mg/dl, sodium of 146 mEq/liter, potassium of 4.6 mEq/liter, chloride of 111 mEq/liter, CO_2 of 10 mEq/liter, blood urea nitrogen of 10 mg/dl, and creatinine of 2.1 mg/dl. George's ethanol level is 200 mg/dl. Liver function tests and a metabolic panel are significant for aspartate aminotransferase (serum glutamic–oxaloacetic transaminase [SGOT]), 414 U (normal at 5–35 U/liter); alanine aminotransferase (serum glutamic–pyruvic transaminase [SGPT]), 6,034 U (normal at 7–56 U/liter); lactate dehydrogenase, 1,753 IU (normal up to 540 U/liter); bilirubin, 0.1 mg/dl; calcium, 9.2 mEq/liter; PO_4, 14.4 mEq/liter; total protein, 5.5; and albumin, 3.1 g/dl. Viral hepatitis serology is negative. The house officer taking care of George is puzzled by the elevation of the serum phosphate level and repeats the blood test. The repeat serum phosphate level is 13.2 mEq/liter.

George does well in the ICU and has no more hypotensive episodes or other complications. He is seen in consultation by a psychiatrist regarding his drug-abuse problem. The next morning, his PO_4 level is 3.4 mEq/liter, calcium is 8.8 mEq/liter, and serum creatinine has returned to normal. SGOT and SGPT go down over the next few days, his chest tube drainage and air leak disappear, and the chest tube is removed. George is discharged home 6 days after admission and follow-up at 2 months is unremarkable.

DISCUSSION

Phosphorus (PO_4) is the major intracellular anion. It is necessary for the metabolism of protein, fat, and carbohydrate, as well as being a source of high-energy chemical bonds and a structural component of phospholipid membranes and nucleic acids. The maintenance of PO_4 homeostasis is primarily under renal control.

Hyperphosphatemia is defined by a serum phosphorus of 4.5 mg/dl or higher. Common causes include a decreased PO_4 excretion (renal failure), increased intracellular to extracellular PO_4 shifts (rhabdomyolysis, sepsis, hypothermia, malignant hyperthermia, tumor chemotherapy), and increased PO_4 ingestion (laxative abuse, enema administration). If untreated, hyperphosphatemia may produce severe hypocalcemia and tetany. Soft tissue calcification and secondary hyperparathyroidism may be the result of long-standing hyperphosphatemia.

Hyperphosphatemia occurs most commonly in patients with renal failure who can not excrete a PO_4 load. Transcellular shift of PO_4 from cells into the extracellular fluid is seen in conditions associated with increased catabolism or tissue destruction (e.g., systemic infections, crush injuries, nontraumatic rhabdomyolysis, hyperthermia, and cytotoxic therapy for malignancies). A high level of PO_4 in and of itself is usually not associated with symptoms even if hyperphosphatemia develops acutely. Hyperphosphatemia may be a contributor to renal insufficiency. However, with rapid elevations of serum PO_4, hypocalcemia and tetany may occur. Serum PO_4 as low as 6 mg/dl may produce symptoms acutely, whereas if that level is reached more slowly, it has no significant effect on serum calcium. Hypocalcemia is the most important short-term consequence of hyperphosphatemia; tetany, neuromuscular hyperexcitability, seizures, and cardiovascular depression may be produced.

In George's case, the presence of very high PO_4 levels can probably be explained by a decrease in oxygen delivery and tissue hypoxia caused by profuse bleeding that resulted in the production of lactic acidosis. Clinically, the presence of acidosis was represented in this case by a change in George's mental status and Kussmaul breathing, as well as by the elevated anion gap.

In 1966, Tranquada et al. reported an association between elevated inorganic PO_4 and lactic acidosis in the presence of tissue hypoxia. This was later confirmed by O'Connor et al. However, in neither of these reports was a relation to an acute hypovolemic episode described. Some authors described an association between hyperphosphatemia and the metabolic acidosis that occurs in cholera. In such cases, high phosphate levels usually fell to normal rapidly after correction of the volume deficit. The hyperphosphatemia seemed to be related to the pH levels and to the renal insufficiency that affects severely dehydrated choleric patients. Phosphorus levels returned to normal more rapidly with treatment than serum creatinine levels. Although no direct explanation for this association was found, it was thought to be related to tissue ischemia and intracellular-extracellular PO_4 shifts caused by acidosis.

It is unlikely that the mild and transient renal insufficiency demonstrated by our patient had any relation to the hyperphosphatemia that occurred. Hyperphosphatemia has not been demonstrated to result from such circumstances.

CLINICAL POINTS TO REMEMBER

1. Hyperphosphatemia may result as a complication of shock.
2. Hyperphosphatemia may produce hypocalcemia that may be clinically significant.
3. Aggressive treatment of shock results in prompt correction of the hyperphosphatemia. Serum calcium and PO_4 levels must be observed carefully.
4. No specific phosphate-lowering treatment is required unless some persistent abnormality (e.g., pre-existing or shock-related azotemia) creates a setting in which a high PO_4 level does not fall promptly.

SELECTED READINGS

Biberstein M, Parker BA. Enema-induced hyper-phosphatemia. Am J Med 1985;79:645–646.

Layon JA, Kirby RR. Fluid and Electrolytes in the Critically Ill. In JM Civetta, RW Taylor, RR Kirby (eds), Critical Care. Philadelphia: Lippincott, 1988;451–474.

O'Connor LR, Klein KL, Bethune JE. Hyperphos-phatemia in lactic acidosis. N Engl J Med 1977;297:707–709.

Slatopolsky E, Rutherford WE, Rosenbaum R, et al. Hyperphosphatemia. Clin Nephrol 1977;7: 138–146.

Tranquada RE, Grant WJ, Peterson CR. Lactic acidosis. Arch Intern Med 1966;117:192–202.

Wason S, Tiler T, Cunha C, et al. Severe hyperphos-phatemia, hypocalcemia, acidosis, and shock in a 5-month-old child following the administration of an adult Fleet enema. Ann Emerg Med 1989;18:696–700.

Index